Immunodeficiencies

Editors

MARK BALLOW
ELENA E. PEREZ

IMMUNOLOGY AND ALLERGY CLINICS OF NORTH AMERICA

www.immunology.theclinics.com

Consulting Editor
LINDA S. COX

August 2020 • Volume 40 • Number 3

ELSEVIER

1600 John F. Kennedy Boulevard • Suite 1800 • Philadelphia, Pennsylvania, 19103-2899
http://www.theclinics.com

IMMUNOLOGY AND ALLERGY CLINICS OF NORTH AMERICA Volume 40, Number 3
August 2020 ISSN 0889-8561, ISBN-13: 978-0-323-76003-4

Editor: Katerina Heidhausen
Developmental Editor: Kristen Helm

Immunology and Allergy Clinics of North America (ISSN 0889–8561) is published quarterly by Elsevier Inc., 360 Park Avenue South, New York, NY 10010-1710. Months of issue are February, May, August, and November. Periodicals postage paid at New York, NY and additional mailing offices. Subscription prices are $344.00 per year for US individuals, $623.00 per year for US institutions, $100.00 per year for US students and residents, $423.00 per year for Canadian individuals, $100.00 per year for Canadian students, $791.00 per year for Canadian institutions, $447.00 per year for international individuals, $791.00 per year for international institutions, $220.00 per year for international students. To receive student/resident rate, orders must be accompanied by name of affiliated institution, date of term, and the *signature* of program/residency coordinator on institution letterhead. Orders will be billed at individual rate until proof of status is received. Foreign air speed delivery is included in all *Clinics* subscription prices. All prices are subject to change without notice. **POSTMASTER**: Send address changes to *Immunology and Allergy Clinics of North America,* Elsevier Health Sciences Division, Subscription Customer Service, 3251 Riverport Lane, Maryland Heights, MO 63043. **Customer Service: 1-800-654-2452 (U.S. and Canada); 314-447-8871 (outside U.S. and Canada). Fax: 314-447-8029. E-mail: journalscustomerservice-usa@elsevier.com (for print support); journalsonlinesupport-usa@elsevier.com (for online support).**

Reprints. For copies of 100 or more, of articles in this publication, please contact the Commercial Reprints Department, Elsevier Inc., 360 Park Avenue South, New York, New York 10010-1710. Tel. 212-633-3874, Fax: 212-633-3820, E-mail: reprints@elsevier.com.

Immunology and Allergy Clinics of North America is covered in MEDLINE/PubMed (Index Medicus), Current Contents/Life Sciences, Science Citation Index, ISI/BIOMED, Chemical Abstracts, and EMBASE/Excerpta Medica.

Contributors

CONSULTING EDITOR

LINDA S. COX, MD, FACP, AAAAI
Department of Medicine and Dermatology, Nova Southeastern University, Casper, Wyoming, USA

EDITORS

MARK BALLOW, MD
Professor, Department of Pediatrics, Division of Allergy and Immunology, Children's Research Institute, Morsani College of Medicine, University of South Florida, Johns Hopkins All Children's Hospital, St Petersburg, Florida, USA

ELENA E. PEREZ, MD, PhD
Partner, Allergy Associates of the Palm Beaches, North Palm Beach, Florida, USA

AUTHORS

CAROLINE ALLAN, MBChB
Department of Virology and Immunology, Auckland City Hospital, Auckland, New Zealand

ROHAN AMERATUNGA, BHB, MBChB, PhD, FRACP, FRCPA, FRCP, FRCPATH, FRCPCH, FFSc, ABMLI
Department of Virology and Immunology, Auckland City Hospital, Associate Professor, Adult and Paediatric Immunologist, Auckland Healthcare Services, Clinical Immunology, Auckland City Hospital, Department of Molecular Medicine and Pathology, Faculty of Medical and Health Sciences, University of Auckland, Auckland, New Zealand

MARK BALLOW, MD
Professor, Department of Pediatrics, Division of Allergy and Immunology, Children's Research Institute, Morsani College of Medicine, University of South Florida, Johns Hopkins All Children's Hospital, St Petersburg, Florida, USA

FRANCISCO A. BONILLA, MD, PhD
Northeast Allergy, Asthma & Immunology, Leominster, Massachusetts, USA

DEEPAK CHELLAPANDIAN, MD, MBBS
Attending Physician, Blood and Marrow Transplant Program, Assistant Professor of Oncology, Johns Hopkins School of Medicine, Johns Hopkins All Children's Hospital, St Petersburg, Florida, USA

MARIA CHITTY-LOPEZ, MD
Fellow in Training, Division of Allergy and Immunology, Department of Pediatrics, University of South Florida, Children's Research Institute, St Petersburg, Florida, USA

CHARLOTTE CUNNINGHAM-RUNDLES, MD, PhD
Professor, Departments of Medicine and Pediatrics, Division of Allergy and Immunology, Icahn School of Medicine at Mount Sinai, New York, New York, USA

CARLA DUFF, CPNP-PC, MSN, APRN, IgCN
Advanced Practice Registered Nurse, Department of Allergy and Immunology, College of Medicine, Adjunct Faculty, College of Nursing, University of South Florida, St Petersburg, Florida, USA

HYE SUN KUEHN, PhD
Immunology Service, Department of Laboratory Medicine, National Institutes of Health (NIH) Clinical Center, Bethesda, Maryland, USA

JENNIFER W. LEIDING, MD
Associate Professor, Division of Allergy and Immunology, Department of Pediatrics, University of South Florida, Children's Research Institute, St Petersburg, Florida, USA

JOAO PEDRO LOPES, MD
Fellow, Departments of Medicine and Pediatrics, Division of Allergy and Immunology, Icahn School of Medicine at Mount Sinai, New York, New York, USA

PAUL J. MAGLIONE, MD, PhD
Assistant Professor, Department of Medicine, Boston University School of Medicine, Boston, Massachusetts, USA

CRISTIANE J. NUNES-SANTOS, MD
Immunology Service, Department of Laboratory Medicine, National Institutes of Health (NIH) Clinical Center, Bethesda, Maryland, USA

ELENA E. PEREZ, MD, PhD
Partner, Allergy Associates of the Palm Beaches, North Palm Beach, Florida, USA

SERGIO D. ROSENZWEIG, MD, PhD
Immunology Service, Department of Laboratory Medicine, National Institutes of Health (NIH) Clinical Center, Bethesda, Maryland, USA

MANDEL SHER, MD
Clinical Professor of Medicine and Pediatrics, Division of Allergy and Immunology, Department of Pediatrics, Morsani College of Medicine, University of South Florida, St. Petersburg, Florida, USA

JACQUELINE D. SQUIRE, MD
Allergy and Immunology Fellow, Division of Allergy and Immunology, Department of Pediatrics, Morsani College of Medicine, University of South Florida, St Petersburg, Florida, USA

SEE-TARN WOON, PhD, FFSc
Department of Virology and Immunology, Auckland City Hospital, Department of Molecular Medicine and Pathology, Faculty of Medical and Health Sciences, University of Auckland, Auckland, New Zealand

Contents

Chronic lung disease is a complication of primary antibody deficiency (PAD) associated with significant morbidity and mortality. Manifestations of lung disease in PAD are numerous. Thoughtful application of diagnostic approaches is imperative to accurately identify the form of disease. Much of the treatment used is adapted from immunocompetent populations. Recent genomic and translational medicine advances have led to specific treatments. As chronic lung disease has continued to affect patients with PAD, we hope that continued advancements in our understanding of pulmonary pathology will ultimately lead to effective methods that alleviate impact on quality of life and survival.

Ikaros zinc finger 1 (IKZF1 or Ikaros) is a hematopoietic zinc finger DNA-binding transcription factor that acts as a critical regulator of lymphocyte and myeloid differentiation. Loss-of-function germline heterozygous mutations in IKZF1 affecting DNA-binding were described as causative of 2 distinct primary immunodeficiency (PID)/inborn error of immunity diseases. Mutations acting by haploinsufficiency present with a common variable immune deficiency-like phenotype mainly characterized by increased susceptibility to infections. Mutations acting in a dominant negative fashion present with a combined immunodeficiency phenotype with high prevalence of Pneumocystis jirovecii pneumonia. Pathophysiology and manifestations of IKAROS-associated diseases in patients with PID are reviewed here.

The number of disorders associated with congenital or acquired asplenia and functional hyposplenism has increased substantially over the past couple decades. Previously, screening for asplenia and hyposplenism was a barrier to identifying patients at risk. Recent methods for measuring splenic function have emerged as accurate and reliable. Identifying patients prevents overwhelming postsplenectomy infection or invasive pneumococcal disease. Approaches to protect patients with asplenia or hyposplenism include patient education of risks and signs/symptoms of infection, vaccination, and antibiotic prophylaxis. Physicians have evaluated methods of preserving splenic function after trauma and sought alternative treatments of refractory cytopenias treated with splenectomy in the past.

Hemophagocytic lymphohistiocytosis (HLH) is a rare but severe form of immune dysregulation often presenting as unremitting fever, cytopenia, hepatosplenomegaly, coagulopathy, and elevation of typical HLH biomarkers. HLH is universally fatal, if left untreated. The HLH-2004 criteria are widely used to diagnose this condition, but there is growing concerns across different settings that its application may result in undertreatment of certain patients. There is an expanding spectrum of genetic conditions that can be complicated by HLH. This review summarizes the current concepts in HLH, the lessons learned from the past, and provide an overview of the latest diagnostic and treatment modalities.

Elena E. Perez and Mark Ballow

Specific antibody deficiency is a primary immunodeficiency disease recognized by the International Union of Immunology Societies and defined by recurrent respiratory infections with normal immunoglobulins, but diminished antibody responses to polysaccharide antigens after vaccination with the 23 valent pneumococcal polysaccharide vaccine. Clinical immunologists struggle with diagnosis and treatment, because the definition of an adequate response to immunization remains controversial. Specific antibody deficiency is managed clinically with close follow-up and prompt treatment of infections, antibiotic prophylaxis, or immune globulin therapy. Treatment is individualized using clinical judgment and existing practice guidelines, which will likely evolve as more studies become available.

Deepak Chellapandian, Maria Chitty-Lopez, and Jennifer W. Leiding

Precision therapy is a concept in which medical treatment is tailored to the patient's individual needs based on individual characteristics and mechanism of disease. Primary immunodysregulatory disorders are an expanding group of primary immunodeficiency diseases that are characterized by early onset autoimmunity and autoinflammation. Precision therapy allows for the alteration of the aberrant immune response leading to clinical improvement of disease related manifestations. This article reviews targeted precision-based therapy for treatment of cytotoxic T-lymphocyte antigen haploinsufficiency, lipopolysaccharide-responsive beige-like anchor deficiency, activated PI3K deficiency syndrome, signal transducer and activator of transcription– 1 and -3 – gain-of-function disorders, and disorders of inflammasome activation.

Carla Duff and Mark Ballow

Immunoglobulin replacement therapy is standard of care in treatment of many primary immunodeficiency diseases. The goal of replacement therapy is to reduce infections in individuals with primary immune deficiency and improve their quality of life. Immunoglobulin replacement therapy is most often lifelong, therefore ease of administration is vital for adherence to treatment. Self-infusion via subcutaneous intravenous immunoglobulin (SCIG) allows patient input to design an individualized and optimal treatment plan. Because SCIG regimens are flexible and allow for increased autonomy, patients receiving SCIG report improved quality of life. This article summarizes the dosing, administration, and adverse event management of SCIG infusions.

IMMUNOLOGY AND ALLERGY CLINICS OF NORTH AMERICA

SERIES OF RELATED INTEREST

Otolaryngologic Clinics
http://oto.theclinics.com/
Medical Clinics
http://medical.theclinics.com/

THE CLINICS ARE AVAILABLE ONLINE!
Access your subscription at:
www.theclinics.com

Preface

Primary Immune Deficiencies: Update on an Evolving Clinical Discipline

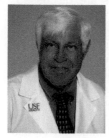
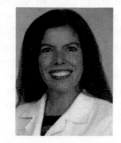

Mark Ballow, MD   Elena E. Perez, MD, PhD
Editors

Every 2 years starting in the 1970s, the International Union of Immunological Societies publishes a list of human inborn errors of immunodeficiency and autoinflammatory disorders. The latest publication in January 2020 lists 416 inborn errors of immunity, including 64 gene defects identified in just the past 2 years since the previous update. The advances in molecular biology, especially next-generation sequencing, have contributed greatly to the rapid identification of novel gene defects. These advances have contributed greatly to our understanding of the immune system, and to a better understanding of the cellular, molecular, and immunologic mechanisms that lead to immune deficiency and autoinflammatory disorders. Clearly these advances translate into better patient diagnosis and novel approaches to therapy. In this issue of *Immunology and Allergy Clinics of North America*, Dr Perez and I have assembled a collection of articles that cover criteria for the diagnosis of immune deficiencies, their laboratory evaluation, and their comorbid conditions and treatment.

Dr Cunningham-Rundles and colleagues are the original creators of the US Immunodeficiency Network (USIDNET), which was created to advance the scientific research of primary immunodeficiency (PI) patients by assembling and maintaining a registry of clinical data. Her contribution together with that of Dr Lopes reviews the history and contributions of the USIDNET registry. The most common antibody immune deficiency is common variable immunodeficiency (CVID).

Immunol Allergy Clin N Am 40 (2020) ix–xi
https://doi.org/10.1016/j.iac.2020.05.001
0889-8561/20/© 2020 Published by Elsevier Inc.

Dating back to the 1980s, and perhaps before, these PIs were referred to as dys-gammaglobulinemia type I, II, and so forth. With the recognition that these PIs were common but variable in presentation, clinical phenotype, and laboratory findings, they were renamed CVID and given criteria for diagnosis. These criteria for diagnosis have evolved over the past 20 years. *Dr Rohan Ameratunga* compares 4 sets of diagnostic criteria for CVID to help clinicians evaluate these complex PI patients. As part of the evaluation of patients for an underlying immune deficiency, vaccines are of critical importance for the diagnosis and management of PI patients. *Dr Tony Bonilla* reviews the concepts of vaccine challenge for evaluating the humoral immune response in PI patients. Current vaccines are discussed, including the diagnostic and therapeutic applications and their important adverse effects. As a follow-up on the topic of CVID, a review by *Dr Paul Maglione* provides a comprehensive review of chronic lung disease in patients with antibody immune deficiency. Several articles are included in this issue on specific PIs. *Dr Sergio Rosenzweig* and colleagues review interesting CVID-like and CID phenotypes of IKAROS-associated diseases due to inborn errors of the *Ikaros/IKZF1* gene, the product of which is a hematopoietic zinc finger DNA-binding transcription factor. *Dr Jacqueline Squire* reviews the evaluation of splenic function to diagnose hypo-splenism and asplenia, the associated clinical presentation of infection in this group of diseases, and management with vaccines and antibiotic prophylaxis. A rare primary immune deficiency that also occurs as a secondary immune deficiency is hemophagocytic lymphohistiocytosis (HLH). *Dr Deepak Chellapandian* reviews the criteria and laboratory diagnosis of this life-threatening hyperinflammatory condition, and the genetics of the primary HLH and the triggers for the secondary causes of HLH. A more common PI that still perplexes clinicians is selective antibody deficiency. *Drs Elena Perez and Mark Ballow* review the criteria, evaluation, and treatment of this interesting PI. Precision therapy is a concept in which medical treatment is tailored to the patient's individual needs based on individual characteristics and mechanism of disease. Primary immuno-dysregulatory disorders (PIRDs) are an expanding group of PI diseases that are characterized by early-onset autoimmunity and autoinflammation. *Dr Jennifer Leiding* and colleagues review the experience with targeted precision-based therapy for the treatment of PIRDs. Mechanism-based therapy using biologics and small-molecule drugs has been very effective at reversing comorbid disease manifestations in PIRDs, offering a most precise therapy for these PI patients. Although subcutaneous immunoglobulin (SCIg) replacement therapy dates back to the 1950s, with the commercial availability of intravenous immunoglobulin in the early 1980s, SCIg therapy has only recently been embraced by the clinical immunology establishment. *Carla Duff and Dr Ballow* review the "nuts and bolts" of SCIg replacement therapy. As SCIg regimens are flexible and allow for increased autonomy, patients receiving SCIg report an improved quality of life. This article summarizes the dosing, administration, and adverse event management of SCIg infusions. The rapidly growing field of primary immune deficiency requires clinical immunologists to stay informed on an array of topics in order to take the best care of our patients. We hope that this collection of reviews serves as a valuable resource for clinical immunologists.

Mark Ballow, MD
Division of Allergy & Immunology
Department of Pediatrics
Morsani College of Medicine
University of South Florida
Children's Research Institute
140 7th Avenue South
CRI 4008
St Petersburg, FL 33701, USA

Elena E. Perez, MD, PhD
840 US Highway 1, Suite 235
North Palm Beach, FL 33408, USA

E-mail addresses:
mballow@usf.edu (M. Ballow)
eperez@pballergy.com (E.E. Perez)

The Importance of Primary Immune Deficiency Registries

The United States Immunodeficiency Network Registry

Joao Pedro Lopes, MD[a,b],
Charlotte Cunningham-Rundles, MD, PhD[a,b],*

KEYWORDS

- Primary immune deficiency • Registry • Immunoglobulin replacement
- Common variable immune deficiency

KEY POINTS

- Patient disease registries are essential data tools for many diseases, but particularly crucial for rare disorders, as most of the primary immune deficiencies.
- The United States Immunodeficiency Network is a research consortium, created to advance the field of primary immune deficiency that includes an extensive registry of patients with primary immune deficiency.
- Multiple points of data analysis have emerged from the registry, generating numerous publications and answering several research questions.

INTRODUCTION

Primary immune deficiencies (PIDs) represent a steadily growing group of more than 400 different disorders caused by defective or absent mutations in genes essential in the immune network. These rare disorders are treatable, in some cases, even curable, once recognized. Without proper recognition and treatment, these defects can be chronic, serious, or even fatal. Because of a general lack of awareness, diagnostic challenges, complexities, and unique differences, the diagnosis of PIDs can be

a Department of Medicine, Division of Allergy and Immunology, Icahn School of Medicine at Mount Sinai, 1425 Madison Avenue, Box 1089, New York, NY 10029, USA; b Department of Pediatrics, Division of Allergy and Immunology, Icahn School of Medicine at Mount Sinai, 1425 Madison Avenue, Box 1089, New York, NY 10029, USA
* Corresponding author. Department of Medicine, Division of Allergy and Immunology, Icahn School of Medicine at Mount Sinai, 1425 Madison Avenue, Box 1089, New York, NY 10029.
E-mail address: charlotte.cunningham-rundles@mssm.edu

Immunol Allergy Clin N Am 40 (2020) 385–402
https://doi.org/10.1016/j.iac.2020.03.002
0889-8561/20/© 2020 Elsevier Inc. All rights reserved.

difficult. Even when recognized, the management of PIDs can be complex. Patient registries are a crucial tool of medical science, as they allow one to gather widespread clinical and laboratory data on selected patient populations that can be used to foster advances in scientific research and ultimately improve patient care. Registries are particularly important for rare diseases, as no one medical center can collect sufficient data to define the actual landscape of these illnesses. From such data, one can estimate the numbers of subjects with these defects, the likely complications, and where new efforts are needed.[1] This was early recognized in PID in many countries, due to the increasing number of these defects, coupled with the extensive clinical and laboratory differences noted between the various conditions. To cope with understanding these genetic defects and their clinical and laboratory features, investigators began using standardized data collection instruments to collect information on patients about 3 decades ago. An early development of a European registry started with an effort in 1994 in Sweden, in collaboration with additional centers in England, Italy, and Spain. This early work compiled limited data on 9707 patients from 26 European countries, creating a basis for research on PID, in particular for clinical studies.[2] Other early efforts in individual countries included Norway,[3] Australia,[4] Spain,[5] Switzerland,[6] and Sweden.[7] The registry started in France in 2005, the Reference Center for PIDs (CEREDIH),[8] is based on a strong network of all university teaching hospitals, with 130 clinicians, 30 diagnostic immunology laboratories, and a dedicated and highly trained staff.

In the United States, realizing the importance of registries in this field, the Immune Deficiency Foundation (IDF) first began collecting data in 1992 under a contract from the National Institutes of Health (NIH) on patients with chronic granulomatous disease (CGD). Subsequently, the contract was extended, and registries were formed to collect data on patients with X-linked agammaglobulinemia (XLA) and X-linked hyper-immunoglobulin M (X-HIGM), common variable immune deficiency (CVID), severe combined immune deficiency (SCID), DiGeorge syndrome (DGS), leukocyte adhesion deficiency, and Wiskott-Aldrich syndrome (WAS).[9] With this as a basis, and the growing realization that these diseases were likely to help elucidate the normal functions of the immune system, the National Institute of Allergy and Infectious Disease and the National Institute of Child Health and Human Development of the NIH posted a competitive research opportunity to build and enhance a PID patient registry, along with other research-enhancing resources. To apply for this research funding, the IDF formed a research program, The United States Immunodeficiency Network (USIDNET) in October 2003. According to its official definition,[9] the USIDNET is "a research consortium established to advance scientific research in the field of PID, by assembling and maintaining a registry of clinical data from patients with PID, providing education and mentoring for young investigators in the field of PI, and acting as a resource for clinical and laboratory research."[10] At the formation of USIDNET, the importance of this kind of unified network between patient registries and clinical immunologists was highlighted in a 2004 editorial.[1] Initially based on paper submissions, with improvements in data capture, a web-based entry system went live in 2008. However, patients still had to participate in the registry via one of the enrolling sites at this time. New funds were obtained in 2013, from the Patient-Centered Outcomes Research Institute initiative, to allow all interested patients in the United States to enroll, and the IDF formed a new means for self-enrollment, called PI CONNECT. In 2016, again to improve data entry, language capture, and data homogeneity, the data migrated to a secure, user-friendly REDCap platform.

Having been supported by the NIH since 2004, the USIDNET registry today contains extensive clinical and laboratory data on more than 7815 patients, with multiple PID diagnoses **(Table 1)**, 37 immune defects, and 2125 identified gene mutations **(Table 2)**. Two thousand six hundred eighty-six have enrolled via the PI CONNECT link. Using the registry data, the IDF and the USIDNET registry have now generated more than 50 publications and more than 50 abstract presentations at national and international conferences. In this paper, the authors review the literature that has been supported by data from the USIDNET registry and how these data have advanced the study and treatment of these diseases.

INSIGHTS FROM THE REGISTRY

One of the first and prominent uses of the registry has been to outline the clinical manifestations, laboratory evaluations, treatments, genetic causes, and outcomes of the individual diseases. Over time, these have resulted in definitive reports on the major disease classifications that have been cited hundreds of times in other publications, including CGD, XLA, HIGM, WAS, SCID, and CVID. These data have also been used to contrast the US patient populations with data registries collected in other countries to determine essential differences in disease ascertainment, microbial differences, treatments, and outcomes. A second main use of the registry has been to answer questions posed by physicians who care for patients. The following outlines the highlights of insights obtained from these many studies.

Chronic Granulomatous Disease

The first data collection formed by the IDF, spearheaded by Dr Jerry Winkelstein, was on subjects with CGD supported by a contract from the NIH. This included 368 patients, the majority (259) with the most common X-linked recessive form, and the rest had autosomal recessive or unknown inheritance forms.[11] This publication was the first to estimate the incidence of CGD in the United States, and it described pneumonia as the most common clinical manifestation (79% of the patients), with Aspergillus infections as the most frequent culprit, followed by suppurative adenitis, subcutaneous and liver abscesses, osteomyelitis, and sepsis. The publication demonstrated the increased mortality rate in the X-linked form, estimated at 5% per year, compared with 2% per year for the recessive form. One goal was to determine the health of these patients: a question brought to the forefront because interferon-gamma (IFN-γ) was an emerging therapy.[12] The high morbidity revealed that better treatments were required. Not surprisingly, these data were referenced the following year by Horwitz and colleagues,[13] who presented the feasibility of nonmyeloablative conditioning followed by T-cell–depleted hematopoietic stem cell allograft transplant as a therapeutic option for patients with CGD with recurrent life-threatening infections and an HLA-identical donor in the family. The data concerning morbidity[11] were referenced by Gallin and colleagues,[14] who designed a randomized, double-blind, placebo-controlled study for fungal infection prophylaxis with itraconazole in patients with CGD. This intended to address the severity of fungal infections that the registry had reported; it demonstrated a clear reduction of frequency of fungal infections in the itraconazole group. Similarly, the morbidity of the original report was cited by Marciano and colleagues[15] when discussing the long-term results of IFN-γ therapy in patients with CGD.

The use of the CGD registry continues: Sacco and colleagues[16] in 2018 examined the prevalence of end-stage renal disease among the patients with CGD in the registry, finding 14 patients with renal disease (2.7% of 516 patients in the database), with 10 of those 14 listed as having renal failure, more than previously described. The current role of allogeneic hematopoietic stem cell transplant (HSCT) among patients with

Table 1
List of primary immune deficiency diagnosis in the USIDNET registry and their frequency (as of January 2020)

Diagnosis	n
Agammaglobulinemia	449
Ataxia telangiectasia	28
Autoimmune lymphoproliferative syndrome (ALPS)	64
Autoinflammatory disease	12
CHARGE syndrome	5
Chronic granulomatous disease	560
Combined immune deficiency	98
Common variable immune deficiency (CVID)	1805
Complement deficiency	26
DiGeorge syndrome	559
Dyskeratosis congenita	2
Ectodermal dysplasia with immunodeficiency (NEMO and others)	30
HLH, including XLP and pigmentary disorders	69
Hyper-IgE syndrome	104
Hyper-IgM syndrome	158
Hypogammaglobulinemia	213
IgA deficiency	72
IgG subclass deficiency	27
Immune deficiency with syndromic features (not otherwise listed)	9
Immune dysregulation	97
Immunodeficiency unknown cause	24
Immunodeficiency with myelodysplasia (GATA2 and others)	68
Interferonopathy (Aicardi–Goutieres syndrome and others)	9
Leukocyte adhesion deficiency	11
Mucocutaneous candidiasis	53
Neutropenia	5
NK cell defect	4
Omenn syndrome	8
Other immune deficiency—known cause	63
Other T-cell problems	8
Predisposition to severe viral infections	30
SCID	355
Specific antibody deficiency with normal Ig concentration and normal number of B cells	99
Susceptibility to mycobacteria (MSMD)	11
TLR pathway abnormality	2
Transient hypogammaglobulinemia of infancy with normal number of B cells	14
Wiskott-Aldrich syndrome	250

Abbreviations: MSMD, Mendelian susceptibility to mycobacterial diseases; NK, natural killer.
   Data from The United States Immunodeficiency Network (USIDNET). Registry-Reported Statistics. Available at: https://usidnet.org/registry-data/stats-registry-enrollment/. Accessed Jan 2020.

Table 2
Frequency of primary immune deficiency diagnostic gene mutation variants in the USIDNET registry (as of January 2020)

Gene Defect	n
11–22 trans/dup at 22q11	1
15q13.3	1
ACAT9	1
ADA	66
AICDA (AID)	3
AIRE	68
AK2 (Hermansky–Pudlak syndrome)	4
ARTEMIS (DCLRE1C)	28
ATM	10
BCL11B	1
BTK	422
C2	14
C3	2
C8	1
CARD11	4
CARD11 (GOF)	3
CARD9	4
CASP10	1
CASP8	2
CBS	1
CD16	2
CD18	1
CD19	3
CD21	1
CD3D	2
CD40 (TNFRSF5)	6
CD40LG	107
CD79a	1
CD86	1
CECR1 (ADA2)	7
Cernunnos (XLF)	2
CFTR	1
CHD7	2
CR2	1
CREBBP	1
CTLA4 (ALPSV)	22
CXCR4	21
CYBA (p22-phox)	31
CYBB (gp91-phox)	357
DAO	1
DEL16q22	1

(continued on next page)

Table 2
(continued)

Gene Defect	n
DEL22q11.2	478
DGCR2	1
DNMT3B (ICF1)	1
DOCK8	27
DQ	1
DUP15q21.1	1
ELANE	1
EPG5	1
F5	1
FOXN1	3
FOXP3 (IPEX)	13
GATA2	66
ICOS	1
IFIH1	1
IFNGR1	9
IFNGR2	1
IFT140	1
IGHM (m heavy chain), PTPRC (CD45)	1
IKBA (NFKIAB)	3
IKBKB	3
IL10	1
IL10RA	2
IL12B (IL-12p40 deficiency)	1
IL12RB1 (IL-12 and IL-23 receptor b1 chain)	3
IL2RA (CD25)	1
IL2RG (gc, CD132)	83
IL7RA	15
IRAK4	1
IRF2BP2	1
ITGB2 (LAD1)	9
JAK3	13
KRAS	1
LIG4	3
LPIN2, RFXAP, TMC8 (EVER2)	1
LRBA	4
LYST (Chediak-Higashi syndrome)	12
MAGT1 (XMEN)	6
MEFV (familial Mediterranean fever)	4
MHC class II	2
MTHFD1	1
MTHFR	2
NCF1 (p47-phox)	76

(continued on next page)

Table 2
(continued)

Gene Defect	n
NCF2 (p67-phox)	14
NEMO (IKBKG)	25
NFKB1	5
NFKB2	5
NLRP3 (NALP3, CIAS1, PYPAF1)	6
OMENN	4
PARN	1
PGM3	2
PIK3CD (PI3 Kinase, GOF)	22
PIK3R1 (PI3 Kinase)	14
PNP	4
PRF1 (FHL2)	2
PRKCD	1
PTPRC (CD45 deficiency)	1
R229 & G319X	1
RAB27A	1
RAD50	1
RAG1	20
RAG2	10
RMRP (CHH)	17
RTEL1	1
SBDS (Shwachman-Diamond syndrome)	1
SERPING1 (C1 inhibitor deficiency)	5
SH2D1A (XLP1)	8
SLC7A7	1
SMARCAL1 (Schimke Immuno-osseous Dysplasia)	2
SMC3	1
SPINK5 (Comel-Netherton syndrome)	4
STAT1	13
STAT1 (GOF)	7
STAT3	50
STAT3 (GOF)	2
STS, WDR1	1
STXBP2 (Munc18–2 deficiency, FHL5)	8
TBX1	1
TLR3	1
TLR9	1
TNFRSF13B (TACI)	32
TNFRSF1A (TRAPS)	1
TNFRSF6 (ALPS-FAS)	9
TRAC (TCR-alpha deficiency)	1
TRNT1	2

(continued on next page)

Table 2 (continued)	
Gene Defect	**n**
TTC37	1
TTC7A	1
TWEAK (TNFSF12)	2
UNC13D (Munc13–4, FHL3)	12
UNG	1
Unspecified	2921
WAS	71
XIAP (BIRC4, XLP2)	15
ZAP70	5

Data from The United States Immunodeficiency Network (USIDNET). Registry-Reported Statistics. Available at: https://usidnet.org/registry-data/stats-registry-enrollment/. Accessed Jan 2020.

CGD in the registry was also recently analyzed by Yonkof and colleagues,[17] who reported 50 out of 507 patients were submitted to transplantation. Patients transplanted before or at the age of 14 years had improved survival.

X-Linked Agammaglobulinemia

A second patient population on which the IDF had early focused was XLA. As early as 1985, in a multicenter retrospective survey of 96 patients, Dr Winkelstein and collaborators had shown the 2 major causes of death in XLA were chronic pulmonary disease leading to cardiac failure and disseminated viral infections, which produced a dermatomyositis-like syndrome, hepatitis, pneumonitis, or meningoencephalitis. Ten years later, with the formation of USIDNET and increased XLA enrollment, Winkelstein and colleagues[18] reported on 201 patients with XLA. The most common clinical presentation was infection (85% of patients); 11% had had neutropenia, which was a known occurrence, but the incidence had not been clarified. There was an average age of diagnosis of 2.6 years in those with an XLA family history (about half of the patients), whereas in its absence, the average age at diagnosis was older at 5.4 years. However, surprisingly, even in those with a known family history, only 34% were diagnosed before developing any symptoms. In this study, over a 4.25-year follow-up, the death rate was 3.75%. One of the known consequences of XLA (and some subjects with CVID) is that live poliovirus formerly used in immunizations could lead to chronic excretion of poliovirus and risk of complications such as chronic meningoencephalitis. In a study that used registry contacts and data, a search for chronic excretors was conducted among 306 patients in the United States, Mexico, Brazil, and the United Kingdom.[19] Fortunately, no excretors were found among this set of studied patients.

What about adults with XLA? Winkelstein used the registry again 2 years later,[20] reporting on 25 patients, and described an increased frequency of hospitalization and missed work or school. However, reassuringly, the patients studied in this report showed a quality of life comparable to the general US population, suggested as possibly due to a higher income and level of education than the general population. This report concluded that, despite the disease impact, patients with XLA could do well.

The loss of immune globulin is compensated in XLA by adequate Ig therapy; for this reason, patients with this immune defect are generally considered to have a low risk of autoimmune or inflammatory disease. However, taking another look at XLA, another recent report using USIDNET data challenges this view. For 149 patients with XLA (average age 17.6 years, range 1–50), the majority (69%) reported having at least one inflammatory symptom. Of these, 28% had been formally diagnosed with an inflammatory condition. 21% reported symptoms of chronic diarrhea, and 17% reported abdominal pain; however, only 4% had been diagnosed with Crohn disease.[21] Perhaps similarly, Barmettler and colleagues[22] examined the frequency of gastrointestinal disease in the patients with XLA in the registry, finding diarrhea to be present intermittently in 38% of the patients, whereas 26% had chronic persistent diarrhea. Abdominal pain was present in 22%, and 9.5% of the USIDNET XLA population had a specific diagnosis of inflammatory bowel disease (IBD) and/or enteritis.

The USIDNET XLA registry data have also been used to elucidate a more global perspective on this immune defect–integrating USIDNET data with registries from other countries. A recent report on 783 patients from 40 centers around the world illustrates both the successes and the challenges for patients and physicians alike.[23] Here, acute and chronic lung diseases accounted for 41% of the deaths. Unusual complications such as IBD and large granular lymphocyte disease, among others, were enumerated. They were individually uncommon but collectively seen in 20.3% of patients. Survival greater than 20 years of age reached greater than 70% in Australia, Europe, and the Americas and was lowest in Africa (22%).

Hyper-IgM Syndrome

Another early data registry collection by the IDF was on the HIGM syndrome. In Italy, data collection on 56 patients with HIGM revealed many severe conditions, including neutropenia in 67%, diarrhea in 55%, sclerosing cholangitis in 19%, neurologic disease and/or unusual and aggressive tumors in 12.5%. All of these were more concerning, as they were more common than anyone center had appreciated.[24] These studies led to work on the inciting causes, cellular mechanisms, and the role of infectious agents and also suggested that HSCT should be considered for treatment.[25] In the United States, Winkelstein and colleagues[26] reported in 2003 on the clinical and immunologic features of 79 patients from 60 unrelated families, all presenting with significant IgG deficiency and most with IgA deficiency, but only about half of the patients with elevated IgM levels showing that, in many ways, the commonly used term "hyper-IgM" was a misnomer. The most common presenting history was infection with pneumonia in 81%, followed by upper respiratory infections (with agents including encapsulated bacteria but also opportunistic organisms such as *Pneumocystis jirovecii*). In contrast to the Italian study, sclerosing cholangitis occurred in 5 (8%) patients and in 4 of these was associated with *Cryptosporidium* infection. The registry of so many patients with this rare condition allowed immunologists to estimate an incidence of this defect in the United States of 1/1,030,000 live births. Based on the reported overall morbidly, Jain and colleagues,[27] seeking new therapies, used these data in their work, seeking a new therapeutic, recombinant CD40 ligand that could lead to partial immune reconstitution in patients with X-HIGM.

In 2016, Leven and colleagues[28] compiled an updated view of patients with HIGM in the registry, then containing 145 patients, almost double the prior reports.[26] Mutations were identified for 85 patients; 82 had a CD40 ligand mutation. The prevalence and types of infections were similar to the 2003 paper, as well as the prevalence of other symptoms, such as diarrhea. The data for the USIDNET cohort suggested a lower incidence of both sclerosing cholangitis and *Cryptosporidium* infection in the US as compared with the European study, possibly due to more recent increased emphasis on *Cryptosporidium* prevention measures such as the use of bottled water.

What about HSCT in HIGM? De la Morena and colleagues[29] examined the long-term outcomes of 176 patients with X-HIGM from several different national and international registries, including USIDNET. These data showed 38% of the patients had been treated with HSCT; however, there was no difference in overall survival between transplant-treated and nontreated patients. Despite that, HSCT patients had an improved quality of life/performance.

Severe Combined Immune Deficiency and Combined Defects

Since the establishment of the registry, one of the central patient populations registered were infants with SCID, as a national resource for infants with these rare conditions was needed for assessment, genetics, and treatment practices. One of the first subsets of patients included were infants with adenosine deaminase (ADA) deficiency. In 2016, 60 patients registered with ADA-deficient SCID, born after 1981, with 85% survival (but none survived with a birth year earlier than 1990). Twenty-three were transplanted; none of these had undergone gene therapy at that time. Using the USID-NET registry data as a resource,[30] Jennifer Puck and the SCID Newborn Screening (NBS) Working Group presented the rationale and strategy for the implementation of a population-based universal NBS for SCID, then implemented with NBS, beginning 2 years later. The USIDNET registry has become a data repository and resource for all infants now discovered in the United States; it will become a crucial tool in the assessment of how newborn discovery will improve survival, with hematopoietic transplant being an early option.[31]

USIDNET data have also been used to compare different countries. Differences in SCID detection in the United States, Middle East, China, Southeast Asia, and Australia were apparent in a 2013 USIDNET report.[32] More recently, Al-Herz and colleagues[33] compared different variables regarding SCID (and combined immune deficiencies) in the USIDNET registry to infants in the Kuwait National PID registry (KNPIDR). The 69 patients with SCID in the KNPIDR were compared with 98 patients from USIDNET, noting the latter presented and were diagnosed at an earlier age. Although based only on the registry data, this study calculated the incidence of SCID/CID in Kuwait to likely be around 8 times higher than in USIDNET. The explanation may reside in the fact that near 70% of these patients in KNIPDR had a family history of PID compared with around 25% in USIDNET. Parental consanguinity greater than 90% was noted, compared with about 10% in the USIDNET data set. HSCT occurred at similar frequencies in both registries, but notably, 51% were matched related in KNIPDR versus 8% in USIDNET.

Common Variable Immune Deficiency

One of the largest collections of data in USIDNET concerns one of the more common and yet diverse of the immune defects, CVID. This resource has been steadily used for many publications over time, reflecting the range of complications that are characteristic of this immune defect. An early report of 700 patients showed that 56% were women; age at diagnosis for men was 25 years and 36 years for women. Complications at that time included infections (88%), autoimmune phenomena (22%; 11% of ITP and 6% of AIHA), and enteropathy (19%). Malignancy was a diagnosis in 13% of the patients, with 6% having a diagnosis of lymphoma. Other findings included bronchiectasis (7%), other chronic lung diseases (11%), splenomegaly (9%), lymphadenopathy (7%), and granulomatous disease (7%).[34] From the same group, Mehra and colleagues[35] used an algorithm to identify 296 chronically ill hospitalized patients with clinical features of immune defects.

With these data as an early baseline, the number of enrolled CVID subjects is now 1805, and it has been used to reexamine the same data points in much greater detail. For example, autoimmune cytopenias were recently reported in 10.2% of patients, with thrombocytopenia (7.4%), anemia (4.5%), and neutropenia (1%). Notably, patients with CVID with any cytopenia were more likely to have additional complications, such as lymphoproliferative disease (including lymphomas), granulomatous disease, liver disease, enteropathy, and interstitial lung disease, as shown, among others, by Feuille and colleagues,[36] confirming the view that immune dysregulation was a common feature with different outcomes. Separately, the rheumatologic manifestations of CVID were characterized by Gutierrez and colleagues.[37] Here, women and nonwhite patients with CVID were more likely to have a rheumatological disease. Lung disease continues to be a significant issue in CVID, and this has been studied in several publications. Weinberger and colleagues[38] compared the pulmonary manifestations between patients with CVID and XLA, finding more asthma, bronchiectasis, interstitial lung disease (ILD), pneumonia, and respiratory infections in the CVID group. Patients with ILD were more likely to have autoimmunity and bronchiectasis. For the patients with CVID, lower levels of T and B cells were observed. This possible association of cellular defects with chronic lung disease in the patients with CVID in the registry was also evaluated by Kellner and colleagues,[39] examining 1518 patients with CVID, comparing 138 (9.1%) who had ILD and 147 (9.7%) who had bronchiectasis, with the 1233 (81.2%) other patients with no reported chronic lung disease. Here also, patients with ILD had lower CD3, CD4, and CD8 cell counts; these patients also had an increased frequency of pneumonia, fungal, and herpes virus infections.

Another way to use USIDNET data is to compare these national data with that of individual medical centers that also collect substantial numbers of patients with PID. Farmer and colleagues[40] have used the resource in this manner, examining noninfectious disease "endotypes" of patients with CVID, by using a method of unbiased network clustering applied to both the USIDNET registry and the Partners data collection in Boston. From that analysis, unique patterns were defined for lymphoproliferative disease (2 clusters, with low class-switched memory B cells and low serum C3 in the total lymphoproliferative cluster), autoimmune disease (2 clusters), and atopic disease (1 cluster, with high serum IgE).

DiGeorge Syndrome

Patel and colleagues[41] published a study in 2012 evaluating the scope of immunoglobulin deficiency in DGS patients from different patient registries, with data from 21 countries, including 1023 patients, 662 of which obtained from the USIDNET Registry. The study concluded an association of DGS with humoral immune deficiency, describing hypogammaglobulinemia in 6% of the patients with DGS in the group who were 3 years old and older, with 3% of the patients in the group requiring intravenous immunoglobulin (IVIG).

Autosomal Dominant Hyper-IgE Syndrome

Gernez and colleagues[42] compiled the data on 85 patients with autosomal dominant hyper-IgE syndrome (AD-HIES) from the USIDNET registry; 45.9% had a family history of AD-HIES. The most common complications were cutaneous abscesses (74.4%), eczema (57.7%), and retained primary teeth (41.4%). The IgE mean level for the group was 8383.7 kU/mL, with eosinophilia present in 49.4%. Prophylactic antimicrobials were used in 56% of the cases for trimethoprim-sulfamethoxazole and 26.6% for antifungal agents; 30.6% of the patients had been placed on immunoglobulin replacement.

ANSWERING QUESTIONS

Physicians who care for subjects with CVID are often asked novel questions about this immune defect that the registry can answer. Since its inception, one of the main goals was to provide a place where such questions could be asked—this is done by using a standard "query" form available on the Internet (https://usidnet.org/registry-data/query-form/). Some of the many questions that have been asked and answered are summarized in the following section.

What Happened to the Patients Infected by Hepatitis C by Contaminated Immunoglobulin Products in 1993 to 1994?

The patients experienced bad outcomes, but physicians did not have the whole story, as it was a matter of litigation. Of 58 PCR-positive hepatitis C–infected patients, 30 were treated with IFN-α, in combination with ribavirin in 5 cases; 26 other subjects were not treated. Of those who were treated, 11 (37%) resolved the infection and became PCR-negative; of the 26 who were not treated, 5 (19%) resolved the infection. Patients aged 20 years or younger had a significantly better outcome compared with those older than age 20 years (P = .02). Five subjects had had liver transplantation, a sixth had had 2 transplants, and 10 (17%) of the group had died.[43]

Do Patients with Primary Immune Deficiency on Intravenous Immunoglobulin Have a Risk of Stroke?

Since the first reports of IVIG-associated thromboembolic events, this question is commonly asked about patients with PID who need this therapy continuously. In fact, all Ig products bear a "black box" warning on the package insert. Basta compared the incidence of stroke among 1127 patients with PID on IVIG from the USIDNET with Centers for Disease Control and Prevention (CDC) data on the frequency of stroke in the general population of the United States. The results showed the overall prevalence of stroke in patients with PID to be approximately 4 times lower than in the general public (0.62 vs 2.6%).[44]

What About Cancer in Primary Immune Deficiency? What Forms and Who Is at Risk?

The question of cancer in the patients with PID in the registry was analyzed by Mayor and colleagues,[45] which showed an overall 1.42-fold increased risk of cancer in these patients when compared with age-adjusted rates from a general population database. Interestingly, women had a similar rate to the general population, with men justifying the increased risk, with a 1.91-fold increase. Most of the increased risk was explained by increases in lymphoma in both genders (10-fold for men, 8.34-fold for women), with common cancers such as lung, colon, breast, and prostate found to have a similar incidence in the registry and the general population.

What About Transplantation Data?

The accumulation of data on the different PID, and the multiple papers originating from it, are a launch pad for future work, with data from different papers arising in registry data, quoted by de la Morena and colleagues[31] when writing up a global review of the advances in transplantation for PID in 2014. That paper comprehensively reviews the remarkable advances in transplantation for patients with both SCID and non-SCID, noting the crucial role of multinational collaborative studies, such as the USIDNET registries, when trying to advance knowledge in the setting of rare disorders.

Who Has Granulomatous Disease in Primary Immune Deficiency and Why?

Leung and colleagues[46] estimated the frequency of granulomas in patients with PID through analyzing both data from the USIDNET registry and commercial insurance and Medicaid databases, with frequencies of 4.4% for USIDNET and of 1.2% to 1.5% in the other databases, with the investigators defining the 1% to 4% range as a baseline to keep in mind for future studies. A landmark study by Perelygina and colleagues,[47] on the same topic of granulomatous disease in PID, also used data from the USIDNET registry. This was the unexpected finding that the granulomatous skin lesions of subjects with significant T-cell defects actually contained Rubella virus, not known until this time.

Do Patients with Primary Immune Deficiency Have Atopic Disease? And If So, Which Ones? What About Drug Allergy?

Patients have asked this question, and there has been no answer thus far. A study[48] found that overall, for 2923 patients, atopic disease and food allergy were less common in PID. Food allergy was reported in CD40 ligand deficiency (7.7%), XLA (7.1%), and hyper-IgE syndrome (HIES) (6.3%) with reactions including anaphylaxis in 20%. Also, atopic dermatitis was most commonly reported in patients with NEMO (62.5%), WAS (41.5%), combined defects (33.3%), selective IgM deficiency (33.3%), and HIES (25%). Patients with CVID, combined defects, and HIES reported both food allergy and atopic dermatitis. Although patients with CVID commonly report this, there is commonly no serum IgE, so is this true? Hartman and colleagues[49] examined 15 patients with CVID at their institution with self-reported penicillin allergy. After skin testing and graded drug challenge, none of the patients had immediate IgE-mediated hypersensitivity to penicillin, which paired with their nondetectable IgE. However, 35% of the CVID subjects in the USIDNET registry had a self-reported diagnosis of drug allergy (specifically beta-lactam allergy in 7%), as compared with a general population self-reported prevalence of 10%.[50] The investigators suggested that true penicillin allergy is likely much lower and needs to be addressed. Amplifying this, Lawrence and colleagues[51] showed that undetectable total serum IgE in 75.6% of the patients with CVID in the registry (compared with only 3.3% in the general population) suggested that the absence of IgE was helpful in the diagnosis of CVID.

Are Children with Common Variable Immune Deficiency Different from Adults with Common Variable Immune Deficiency?

Sanchez and colleagues[52] compared registry data on pediatric and adult patients with CVID and found few differences suggesting that this was more of a continuum; however, as one would expect, there was an increased frequency of otitis media and failure to thrive in the children. Looking at this from another standpoint, Yong and colleagues[53] assessed the immunologic and phenotypic associations of different levels of switched memory B cells in the pediatric CVID population.

What Are the Quality of Life and Perceived Health in Primary Immune Deficiency? What About Fatigue? What About Being Underweight?

Seeborg and colleagues[54] published data on perceived health of 1587 patients with PID, respondents to a national survey using the IDF database registry, using data from the USIDNET registry to compare the study demographics with other PID registries, finding a similar average age of 30 years. Patients with immune defects commonly say that they are overly fatigued, and this is a significant issue in their lives. To examine this, Hajjar and colleagues[55] queried the USIDNET registry data. Although 18% of the patients reported fatigue, as compared with a population prevalence of around 6% to 7.5%, those with primary antibody diseases (particularly CVID) had higher levels of fatigue, with 69% of the patients in this group reporting this. Ruffner and colleagues[56] looked specifically at underweight patients with PID in the USIDNET registry, finding granulomatous disease and earlier age of CVID diagnosis associated with the presence of underweight in the adult population. At the same time, for the pediatric population, underweight patients with CVID were associated with the presence of lymphopenia. The investigators also looked into the prevalence of obesity in the registry, which was similar to the general population.

What Does the Registry Tell Us About the Use of Immune Globulin Products in the United States?

Stonebraker and colleagues[57] examined data regarding the dosage of immunoglobulin replacement therapy used by USIDNET registry patients as compared with the medical literature and other databases. The investigators concluded that significantly different doses of immunoglobulin are used in different locations to treat patients with CVID, and concluded also that different doses are used when comparing patients with CVID with patient with XLA. They noted that an estimate of the latent therapeutic demand for each country would help to define what an adequate product supply for subjects with PID is.

SUMMARY

As seen earlier, the human, financial, and time investment placed in the creation of a project such as the USIDNET registry has had a significant impact on scientific advancements and understanding of PID as a whole, as well as of specific diseases. Naturally, the quantity and quality of the data in a registry depend on a constant addition of new data and maintenance/cleaning of the existing data, to guarantee the growth in knowledge does not plateau or, even worse, decrease. Data collection can reveal areas of low-diagnostic rates and potentially the lengths of diagnostic delay, commonly associated with increased morbidity and mortality. In fact, such regional differences were noted in the French registry.[8] Patient registries provide information helpful to funding agencies and governmental bodies to plan educational programs and estimate treatments and their long-term costs. These data are also crucial to the Pharmaceutical Industry to plan for the supplies of medical products and to seek new areas of research.[58] Patients are essential stakeholders in this work, and for this reason, the IDF and PICONNECT, providing a means for patient enrollment of valuable and verified data, have been an essential ingredient of USIDNET. As the discovery of specific monogenic diseases and better understanding and definition of polygenic diseases has been growing at a fast pace and will tend to grow exponentially in the next decades, it is crucial that an excellent database of clinical data and a biorepository of patient samples pairs with all the information added by genetic studies. Continuing this process, expanding on it, and refining it will benefit us all as a scientific community, but, even more importantly, it will benefit our patients, reinforcing our goal of continually improving their quantity and quality of life.

DISCLOSURE

This work was supported by the National Institutes of Health, AI-101093, AI-086037, AI-48693, and the David S Gottesman Immunology Chair.

REFERENCES

1. Shearer WT, Cunningham-Rundles C, Ochs HD. Primary immunodeficiency: looking backwards, looking forwards. J Allergy Clin Immunol 2004;113(4):607–9.
2. Eades-Perner AM, Gathmann B, Knerr V, et al. The European internet-based patient and research database for primary immunodeficiencies: results 2004-06. Clin Exp Immunol 2007;147(2):306–12.
3. Stray-Pedersen A, Abrahamsen TG, Froland SS. Primary immunodeficiency diseases in Norway. J Clin Immunol 2000;20(6):477–85.
4. Baumgart KW, Britton WJ, Kemp A, et al. The spectrum of primary immunodeficiency disorders in Australia. J Allergy Clin Immunol 1997;100(3):415–23.
5. Matamoros NF, Mila JM, Llambi T, et al. Primary immunodeficiency syndrome in Spain: first report of the national registry in children and adults. J Clin Immunol 1997;17:333–9.
6. Ryser O, Morell A, Hitzig WH. Primary immunodeficiencies in Switzerland: first report of the national registry in adults and children. J Clin Immunol 1988;8(6): 479–85.
7. Fasth A. Primary immunodeficiency disorders in Sweden: cases among children, 1974-1979. J Clin Immunol 1982;2(2):86–92.
8. CEREDIH: The French PID study group. The French national registry of primary immunodeficiency diseases. Clin Immunol 2010;135(2):264–72.
9. USIDNETmission. Available at: https://usidnet.org/usidnet-mission/. Accessed December 8, 2019.
10. Sullivan KE, Puck JM, Notarangelo LD, et al. USIDNET: a strategy to build a community of clinical immunologists. J Clin Immunol 2014;34(4):428–35.
11. Winkelstein JA, Marino MC, Johnston RB Jr, et al. Chronic granulomatous disease. Report on a national registry of 368 patients. Medicine (Baltimore) 2000; 79(3):155–69.
12. Gallin JI. Interferon-gamma in the management of chronic granulomatous disease. Rev Infect Dis 1991;13(5):973–8.
13. Horwitz ME, Barrett AJ, Brown MR, et al. Treatment of chronic granulomatous disease with nonmyeloablative conditioning and a T-cell-depleted hematopoietic allograft. N Engl J Med 2001;344(12):881–8.
14. Gallin JI, Alling DW, Malech HL, et al. Itraconazole to prevent fungal infections in chronic granulomatous disease. N Engl J Med 2003;348(24):2416–22.
15. Marciano BE, Wesley R, De Carlo ES, et al. Long-term interferon-gamma therapy for patients with chronic granulomatous disease. Clin Infect Dis 2004;39(5): 692–9.
16. Sacco KA, Garabedian E, Sullivan KE, et al. Renal disease in chronic granulomatous disease: data from the USIDNETregistry. J Clin Immunol 2018;38(5):556–7.
17. Yonkof JR, Gupta A, Fu P, et al, the United States Immunodeficiency Network C. Role of allogeneic hematopoietic stem cell transplant for Chronic Granulomatous Disease (CGD): a Report of the United States Immunodeficiency Network. J Clin Immunol 2019;39(4):448–58.
18. Winkelstein JA, Marino MC, Lederman HM, et al. X-linked agammaglobulinemia: report on a United States registry of 201 patients. Medicine 2006;85(4):193–202.
19. Halsey NA, Pinto J, Espinosa-Rosales F, et al. Search for poliovirus carriers among people with primary immune deficiency diseases in the United States, Mexico, Brazil, and the United Kingdom. Bull WorldHealthOrgan 2004;82(1):3–8.
20. Winkelstein JA, Conley ME, James C, et al. Adults with X-linked agammaglobulinemia: impact of disease on daily lives, quality of life, educational and

socioeconomic status, knowledge of inheritance, and reproductive attitudes. Medicine 2008;87(5):253–8.

21. Hernandez-Trujillo VP, Scalchunes C, Cunningham-Rundles C, et al. Autoimmunity and inflammation in X-linked agammaglobulinemia. J Clin Immunol 2014; 34(6):627–32.

22. Barmettler S, Otani IM, Minhas J, et al. Gastrointestinal Manifestations in X-linked Agammaglobulinemia. J Clin Immunol 2017;37(3):287–94.

23. El-Sayed ZA, Abramova I, Aldave JC, et al. X-linked agammaglobulinemia (XLA):phenotype, diagnosis, and therapeutic challenges around the world. WorldAllergyOrgan J 2019;12(3):100018.

24. Levy J, Espanol-Boren T, Thomas C, et al. Clinical spectrum of X-linked hyper-IgM syndrome. J Pediatr 1997;131(1 Pt 1):47–54.

25. Hayward AR, Levy J, Facchetti F, et al. Cholangiopathy and tumors of the pancreas, liver, and biliary tree in boys with X-linked immunodeficiency with hyper-IgM. J Immunol 1997;158(2):977–83.

26. Winkelstein JA, Marino MC, Ochs H, et al. The X-linked hyper-IgM syndrome: clinical and immunologic features of 79 patients. Medicine 2003;82(6):373–84.

27. Jain A, Kovacs JA, Nelson DL, et al. Partial immune reconstitution of X-linked hyper IgM syndrome with recombinant CD40 ligand. Blood 2011;118(14):3811–7.

28. Leven EA, Maffucci P, Ochs HD, et al. Hyper IgM Syndrome: a report from the USIDNETregistry. J Clin Immunol 2016;36(5):490–501.

29. de la Morena MT, Leonard D, Torgerson TR, et al. Long-term outcomes of 176 patients with X-linked hyper-IgM syndrome treated with or without hematopoietic cell transplantation. J Allergy Clin Immunol 2017;139(4):1282–92.

30. Puck JM, Group SNSW. Population-based newborn screening for severe combined immunodeficiency: steps toward implementation. The J Allergy Clin Immunol 2007;120(4):760–8.

31. de la Morena MT, Nelson RP Jr. Recent advances in transplantation for primary immune deficiency diseases: a comprehensive review. Clin Rev Allergy Immunol 2014;46(2):131–44.

32. Al-Herz W, Al-Mousa H. Combined immunodeficiency: the Middle East experience. J Allergy Clin Immunol 2013;131(3):658–60.

33. Al-Herz W, Notarangelo LD, Sadek A, et al. Combined immunodeficiency in the United States and Kuwait: comparison of patients' characteristics and molecular diagnosis. Clin Immunol 2015;161(2):170–3.

34. Cunningham-Rundles C, Knight AK. Common variable immune deficiency: reviews, continued puzzles, and a new registry. Immunol Res 2007;38(1–3):78–86.

35. Mehra A, Sidi P, Doucette J, et al. Subspecialty evaluation of chronically ill hospitalized patients with suspected immune defects. Ann Allergy Asthma Immunol 2007;99(2):143–50.

36. Feuille EJ, Anooshiravani N, Sullivan KE, et al. Autoimmune cytopenias and associated conditions in CVID: a report from the USIDNETregistry. J Clin Immunol 2018;38(1):28–34.

37. Gutierrez MJ, Sullivan KE, Fuleihan R, et al. Phenotypic characterization of patients with rheumatologic manifestations of common variable immunodeficiency. Semin Arthritis Rheum 2018;48(2):318–26.

38. Weinberger T, Fuleihan R, Cunningham-Rundles C, et al. Factors beyond lack of antibody govern pulmonary complications in primary antibody deficiency. J Clin Immunol 2019;39(4):440–7.

39. Kellner ES, Fuleihan R, Cunningham-Rundles C, et al. Cellular defects in CVID patients with chronic lung disease in the USIDNETregistry. J Clin Immunol 2019;39(6):569–76.

40. Farmer JR, Ong MS, Barmettler S, et al. Common variable immunodeficiency non-infectious disease endotypes redefined using unbiased network clustering in large electronic datasets. Front Immunol 2017;8:1740.

41. Patel K, Akhter J, Kobrynski L, et al. Immunoglobulin deficiencies: the B-lymphocyte side of DiGeorge Syndrome. J Pediatr 2012;161(5):950–3.

42. Gernez Y, Freeman AF, Holland SM, et al. Autosomal dominant Hyper-IgE syndrome in the USIDNETregistry. J Allergy Clin Immunol Pract 2018;6(3):996–1001.

43. Razvi S, Schneider L, Jonas MM, et al. Outcome of intravenous immunoglobulin-transmitted hepatitis C virus infection in primary immunodeficiency. Clin Immunol 2001;101(3):284–8.

44. Basta M. Intravenous immunoglobulin-related thromboembolic events - an accusation that proves the opposite. Clin Exp Immunol 2014;178(Suppl 1):153–5.

45. Mayor PC, Eng KH, Singel KL, et al. Cancer in primary immunodeficiency diseases: cancer incidence in the United States Immune Deficiency Network Registry. J Allergy Clin Immunol 2018;141(3):1028–35.

46. Leung J, Sullivan KE, Perelygina L, et al. Prevalence of granulomas in patients with primary immunodeficiency disorders, united states: data from National Health Care Claims and the US Immunodeficiency Network Registry. J Clin Immunol 2018;38(6):717–26.

47. Perelygina L, Plotkin S, Russo P, et al. Rubella persistence in epidermal keratinocytes and granuloma M2 macrophages in patients with primary immunodeficiencies. J Allergy Clin Immunol 2016;138(5):1436–1439 e1411.

48. Tuano KS, Orange JS, Sullivan K, et al. Food allergy in patients with primary immunodeficiency diseases: prevalence within the US Immunodeficiency Network (USIDNET). J Allergy Clin Immunol 2015;135(1):273–5.

49. Hartman H, Schneider K, Hintermeyer M, et al. Lack of clinical hypersensitivity to penicillin antibiotics in common variable immunodeficiency. J Clin Immunol 2017;37(1):22–4.

50. Joint Task Force on Practice Parameters, American Academy of Allergy, Asthma and Immunology, American College of Allergy, Asthma and Immunology, Joint Council of Allergy, Asthma and Immunology. Drug allergy: an updated practice parameter. Ann Allergy Asthma Immunol 2010;105(4):259–73.

51. Lawrence MG, Palacios-Kibler TV, Workman LJ, et al. Low serum IgE is a sensitive and specific marker for Common Variable Immunodeficiency (CVID). J Clin Immunol 2018;38(3):225–33.

52. Sanchez LA, Maggadottir SM, Pantell MS, et al. Two sides of the same coin: pediatric-onset and adult-onset common variable immune deficiency. J Clin Immunol 2017;37(6):592–602.

53. Yong PL, Orange JS, Sullivan KE. Pediatric common variable immunodeficiency: immunologic and phenotypic associations with switched memory B cells. Pediatr Allergy Immunol 2010;21(5):852–8.

54. Seeborg FO, Seay R, Boyle M, et al. Perceived health in patients with primary immune deficiency. J Clin Immunol 2015;35(7):638–50.

55. Hajjar J, Guffey D, Minard CG, et al. Increasedincidence of fatigue in patients with primary immunodeficiency disorders: prevalence and associations within the US immunodeficiency network registry. J Clin Immunol 2017;37(2):153–65.

56. Ruffner MA, Group UBW, Sullivan KE. Complications associated with under-weight primary immunodeficiency patients: prevalence and associations within the USIDNET Registry. J Clin Immunol 2018;38(3):283–93.
57. Stonebraker JS, Hajjar J, Orange JS. Latent therapeutic demand model for the immunoglobulin replacement therapy of primary immune deficiency disorders in the USA. Vox Sang 2018;113:430–40.
58. Chapel H, Prevot J, Gaspar HB, et al. Primary immune deficiencies - principles of care. Front Immunol 2014;5:627.

Defining Common Variable Immunodeficiency Disorders in 2020

Rohan Ameratunga, BHB, MBChB, PhD, FRACP, FRCPA, FRCP, FRCPATH, FRCPCH, FFSc, ABMLI[a,b,c,d,*], Caroline Allan, MBChB[a], See-Tarn Woon, PhD, FFSc[a,d]

KEYWORDS

- Common variable immunodeficiency • Diagnostic criteria • HGUS • THA • CVID
- SCIG • IVIG • Hypogammaglobulinemia

KEY POINTS

- The causes of common variable immunodeficiency disorders (CVID) are by definition unknown at this time.
- All current diagnostic criteria for CVID mandate exclusion of known causes of hypogammaglobulinemia.
- If a causative defect is identified, patients are removed from the umbrella diagnosis of CVID and are reclassified as having a CVID-like disorder.
- The understanding of these disorders is continuing to evolve and several recent studies have examined some of these areas of uncertainty.

INTRODUCTION

Common variable immunodeficiency disorders (CVIDs) are the most frequent symptomatic primary immune deficiencies (PIDs) in adults. Most patients suffer recurrent infections as a consequence of immune system failure (ISF) caused by late-onset antibody failure.[1–4] A significant minority of patients with CVID also have an increased risk of autoimmune or inflammatory disorders because of immune dysregulation. Although many patients have symptoms dating back to infancy,[5] most are diagnosed beyond early childhood.

a Department of Virology and Immunology, Auckland City Hospital, Auckland, New Zealand; b Auckland Healthcare Services, Park Road, Grafton, Auckland 1010, New Zealand; c Clinical Immunology, Auckland City Hospital, Auckland, New Zealand; d Department of Molecular Medicine and Pathology, Faculty of Medical and Health Sciences, University of Auckland, Auckland, New Zealand
* Corresponding author. Auckland Healthcare Services, Park Road, Grafton, Auckland 1010, New Zealand.
E-mail address: rohana@adhb.govt.nz

Immunol Allergy Clin N Am 40 (2020) 403–420
https://doi.org/10.1016/j.iac.2020.03.001
0889-8561/20/© 2020 Elsevier Inc. All rights reserved.

immunology.theclinics.com

Most of the adult patients with CVID have immunoglobulin G (IgG) levels less than 5 g/L (nr = 7–14).[6] Most patients also have reduced or undetectable IgA and/or IgM levels.[1,7] Other laboratory features include impaired switched memory B cells and increased numbers of CD21 (low) B cells in the periphery.[8] A subgroup of patients with concomitant severe T-cell defects are defined separately as late-onset combined immune deficiency (LOCID),[9] although there is an argument that these patients should remain in one of the overlapping subphenotypes of CVID and CVID-like disorders.[10]

In addition to the laboratory abnormalities outlined earlier, many patients have characteristic histologic lesions, including nodular lymphoid hyperplasia of the gut, nodular regenerative hyperplasia of the liver, and a granulomatous disorder, often associated with lymphoid interstitial pneumonitis of the lungs, termed granulomatous lymphocytic interstitial lung disease (GLILD).[11,12] Markedly reduced or absent plasma cells in gastrointestinal and lymph node biopsies are another characteristic feature in most of the patients with CVID.[13]

SEPARATION OF COMMON VARIABLE IMMUNODEFICIENCY DISORDERS AND COMMON VARIABLE IMMUNODEFICIENCY DISORDERS-LIKE DISORDERS IS BASED ON GENETICS

Over the last 17 years, approximately 40 genetic defects have been identified in patients with a CVID phenotype.[14] If the genetic variant (mutation) causes the disorder (*NFKB1, NFKB2* etc.), patients are removed from the broad umbrella diagnosis of CVID and are stated to have a CVID-like disorder, caused by a specific PID/inborn error of immunity (IEI).[15] Currently, a causative mutation can be identified in approximately 25% of patients with a CVID phenotype, in nonconsanguineous populations.[16] In addition to monogenic defects, we have recently described a patient with a causative digenic disorder resulting from epistatic interactions of the TACI (*TNFRSF13B*) and *TCF3* genes leading to a severe CVID-like disorder.[17] Epistasis is the synergistic, nonlinear interaction of 2 or more genetic loci leading to either a much more severe disorder or a completely different phenotype.[18]

All current definitions of CVID exclude patients with a known disorder, which is the basis for separating patients with a causative mutation, from those who do not. In contrast, other genetic variants, including TACI (*TNFRSF13B*), BAFFR (*TNFRSF13C*), TWEAK (*TNFSF12*), *MSH5*, and TRAIL (*TNFSF10*) predispose to or modify disease severity.[17] Mutations of TACI (*TNFRSF13B*), BAFFR (*TNFRSF13C*), TWEAK (*TNFSF12*), *MSH5*, and TRAIL (*TNFSF10*) are found in healthy individuals, at a much higher frequency than the lifetime incidence of CVID.[19,20] Patients bearing these variants thus remain within the definition of CVID, as they do not have causative mutations.

COMMON VARIABLE IMMUNODEFICIENCY DISORDERS DIAGNOSTIC CRITERIA

Soon after primary immunodeficiency disorders were first identified, it became apparent that there were several mostly adult patients who had predominant antibody deficiency. In 1971, the term "common variable immunodeficiency" was applied to this group of patients.

Because the cause of these disorders is unknown, diagnostic criteria play an important role in identifying these patients, so they can receive appropriate treatment. Subcutaneous immunoglobulin or intravenous immunoglobulin (SCIG/IVIG) replacement can substantially improve both quality of life and longevity of patients with CVID. This underscores the importance of precise diagnostic criteria for CVID.[21]

Over the last 2 decades, there have been efforts to formulate diagnostic criteria to better define this heterogeneous group of disorders. Here we compare the original ESID/Pan American Group for Immune Deficiency (PAGID, 1999) criteria, the Ameratunga and colleagues (2013) criteria, the revised ESID registry (2014) criteria, and the most recent CVID international consensus (ICON) (2016) criteria (**Boxes 1–4**). The understanding of CVID continues to evolve and we present our perspective of these criteria.

The ESID/PAGID (1999) Criteria for Common Variable Immunodeficiency Disorders

The ESID/PAGID (1999) criteria stated CVID was a diagnosis of exclusion (see **Box 1**).[22] Patients were required to have an IgG level less than 7 g/L (2 SD less than the mean, or more accurately, less than the 97.5th percentile, because Ig levels do not follow a Gaussian distribution[23]), as well as impaired vaccine challenge responses or absent isohemagglutinins. Patients were also required to have a reduction of either IgM or IgA and other secondary causes of hypogammaglobulinemia were to be excluded. It was believed that these criteria were relatively simple and could be applied to diagnose patients with CVID in developing countries.

The major limitation of the ESID/PAGID (1999) criteria was the difficulty in interpretation of vaccine challenge responses, which are a pivotal component of these criteria (**Box 5**). These criteria did not specify which vaccines should be used or the threshold for identifying vaccine failure. Therefore, asymptomatic patients with trivial hypogammaglobulinemia with mildly impaired diphtheria antibody responses could be classified as having CVID. Poor responses to the diphtheria vaccine are common, even in normal persons, particularly with advancing age.[24] Several eminent investigators expressed concern about the need for revised diagnostic criteria for CVID.[25,26]

Box 1
The original ESID/PAGID (1999) criteria for probable and possible common variable immunodeficiency disorders

Probable
  Probable CVID
    Male or female patient who has a marked decrease of IgG (at least 2 SD less than the mean for age) and a marked decrease in at least one of the isotypes IgM or IgA and fulfills all of the following criteria:
    1. Onset of immunodeficiency at age older than 2 years
    2. Absent isohemagglutinins and/or poor response to vaccines
    3. Defined causes of hypogammaglobulinemia have been excluded
  Possible CVID
    Male or female patient who has a marked decrease (at least 2 SD less than the mean for age) in at least one of the major isotypes (IgM, IgG, and IgA) and fulfills all of the following criteria:
    1. Onset of immunodeficiency at age older than 2 years
    2. Absent isohemagglutinins and/or poor response to vaccines
    3. Defined causes of hypogammaglobulinemia have been excluded

From Conley ME, Notarangelo LD, Etzioni A. Diagnostic criteria for primary immunodeficiencies. Representing PAGID (Pan-American Group for Immunodeficiency) and ESID (European Society for Immunodeficiencies). Clin Immunol 1999;93(3):191; with permission.

Box 2
New diagnostic criteria for common variable immunodeficiency disorders

A. Must meet all major criteria
   - Hypogammaglobulinemia IgG less than 5 g/L[6]
   - No other cause identified for immune defect
   - Age greater than 4 years

B. Sequelae directly attributable to immune system failure (ISF) (1 or more)
   - Recurrent, severe, or unusual infections
   - Poor response to antibiotics
   - Breakthrough infections in spite of prophylactic antibiotics
   - Infections in spite of appropriate vaccination, for example, HPV disease
   - Bronchiectasis and/or chronic sinus disease
   - Inflammatory disorders or autoimmunity

C. Supportive laboratory evidence (3 or more criteria)
   - Concomitant reduction or deficiency of IgA (<0.8 g/L) and/or IgM (0.4 g/L)[1,3]
   - Presence of B cells but reduced memory B-cell subsets and/or increased CD21 low subsets by flow cytometry[8]
   - IgG3 deficiency (<0.2 g/L)[38,39]
   - Impaired vaccine responses compared with age-matched controls[55]
   - Transient vaccine responses compared with age-matched controls[20,36]
   - Absent isohemagglutinins (if not blood group AB)
   - Serologic evidence of significant autoimmunity, for example, Coombes test
   - Sequence variations of genes predisposing to CVID, for example, *TACI, BAFFR, MSH5* etc.[19]

D. Presence of relatively specific histologic markers of CVID (not required for diagnosis but presence increases diagnostic certainty, in the context of Category A and B criteria)
   - Lymphoid interstitial pneumonitis
   - Granulomatous disorder[11,12]
   - Nodular regenerative hyperplasia of the liver[56,57]
   - Nodular lymphoid hyperplasia of the gut
   - Absence of plasma cells on gut biopsy[13]

Meeting criteria in categories ABC or ABD indicates probable CVID. Patients meeting criteria ABC and ABD should be treated with IVIG/SCIG (see **Fig. 1**). Patients meeting criteria A alone, AB or AC or AD but not B, are termed possible CVID. Some of these patients may need to be treated with IVIG/SCIG. Patients with IgG levels greater than 5 g/L, not meeting any other criteria are termed hypogammaglobulinemia of uncertain significance (HGUS). These diagnostic criteria must be applied sequentially, as none are specific individually.

Adapted from Ameratunga R, Woon ST, Gillis D, et al. New diagnostic criteria for common variable immune deficiency (CVID), which may assist with decisions to treat with intravenous or subcutaneous immunoglobulin. Clin Exp Immunol 2013;174(2):205; with permission.

Ameratunga and Colleagues (2013) Diagnostic Criteria for Common Variable Immunodeficiency Disorders

Seven years ago, we published new diagnostic criteria for possible or probable CVID (Ameratunga and colleagues[21] 2013, **Box 2**), based on peer-reviewed literature. Because the etiology of these conditions is unknown, we did not think it was possible to make a definite diagnosis of CVID. Treatment recommendations were closely linked to these diagnostic criteria (**Fig. 1**).[27] The Ameratunga and colleagues[28] (2013) criteria emphasized both the clinical sequelae and laboratory abnormalities of ISF in these patients.

We set a threshold less than 5 g/L for IgG for adults, as this was the cutoff in the French CVID study.[6] Patients were required to be older than 4 years and should not

---

Box 3
Revised ESID registry (2014) criteria for common variable immunodeficiency disorders

ESID Registry criteria 2019

At least one of the following:
- Increased susceptibility to infection
- Autoimmune manifestations
- Granulomatous disease
- Unexplained polyclonal lymphoproliferation
- Affected family member with antibody deficiency

AND marked decrease of IgG and marked decrease of IgA with or without low IgM levels (measured at least twice; <2SD of the normal levels for their age)

AND at least one of the following:
- Poor antibody response to vaccines (and/or absent isohemagglutinins), that is, absence of
- Protective levels despite vaccination where defined
- Low switched memory B cells (<70% of age-related normal value)

AND secondary causes of hypogammaglobulinemia have been excluded (eg, infection, protein loss, medication, malignancy)

AND diagnosis is established after the fourth year of life (but symptoms may be present before)

AND no evidence of profound T-cell deficiency, defined as 2 of the following (one-fourth years of life):
- CD4 numbers/microliter: 2 to 6 y < 300, 6 to 12 y < 250, older than 12 y < 200
- % naïve of CD4: 2 to 6 y < 25%, 6 to 16 y < 20%, older than 16 y < 10%
- T-cell proliferation absent

ESID unclassified antibody deficiency (UCH)

At least one of the following:
- Recurrent or severe bacterial infections
- Autoimmune phenomena (especially cytopenias)
- Polyclonal lymphoproliferation
- Affected family member

AND at least one of the following:
- Marked decrease of at least one of total IgG, IgG1, IgG2, IgG3, IgA, or IgM levels
- Failure of IgG antibody response to vaccines

AND secondary causes of hypogammaglobulinemia have been excluded (eg, infection, protein loss, medication, malignancy)

AND no clinical signs of T-cell–related disease

AND does not fit any of the other working definitions (excluding "unclassified immunodeficiencies")

Adapted from Seidel MG, Kindle G2, Gathmann B, et al. The European Society for Immunodeficiencies (ESID) Registry Working Definitions for the Clinical Diagnosis of Inborn Errors of Immunity. J Allergy Clin Immunol Pract 2019;7(6):1766; with permission.

---

have a known cause for their hypogammaglobulinemia. The most important feature of these criteria was clinical evidence of ISF (Category B). Patients must have predisposition to infections and/or autoimmune disease, as a direct result of their immune system failure. The intention was to distinguish symptomatic patients from those who were well, who we predicted would have a different prognostic trajectory. These symptomatic patients must have relevant laboratory evidence of ISF or dysfunction (Category C) or the characteristic histologic findings (Category D) associated with CVID (see **Box 2**).

Box 4
ICON (2016) criteria for common variable immunodeficiency disorders

Consensus definition of CVID (ICON) 2016

1. Most patients will have at least one of the characteristic clinical manifestations (infection, autoimmunity, lymphoproliferation). However, a diagnosis of CVID may be conferred on asymptomatic individuals who fulfill criteria 2 to 5, especially in familial cases.
2. Hypogammaglobulinemia should be defined according to the age-adjusted reference range for the laboratory in which the measurement is performed. The IgG level must be repeatedly low in at least 2 measurements more than 3 weeks apart in all patients. Repeated measurement may be omitted if the level is very low (<100–300 mg/dL depending on age), other characteristic features are present, and it is considered in the best interest of the patient to initiate therapy with IgG as quickly as possible.
3. IgA or IgM level must also be low. (Note that some experts prefer a more narrow definition requiring low IgA level in all patients.)
4. It is strongly recommended that all patients with an IgG level of more than 100 mg/dL should be studied for responses to T-dependent (TD) and T-independent (TI) antigens, whenever possible. In all patients undergoing such testing, there must be a demonstrable impairment of response to at least 1 type of antigen (TD or TI). At the discretion of the practitioner, specific antibody measurement may be dispensed with if all other criteria are satisfied and if the delay incurred by prevaccination and postvaccination antibody measurement is thought to be deleterious to the patient's health.
5. Other causes of hypogammaglobulinemia must be excluded (see **Box 1**).
6. Genetic studies to investigate monogenic forms of CVID or for disease-modifying polymorphisms are not generally required for diagnosis and management in most of the patients, especially those who present with infections only without immune dysregulation, autoimmunity, malignancy, or other complications. In these latter groups of patients, however, single gene defects may be amenable to specific therapies (eg, stem cell therapy) and molecular genetic diagnosis should be considered when possible.

From Bonilla FA, Barlan I, Chapel H, et al. International Consensus Document (ICON): Common Variable Immunodeficiency Disorders. J Allergy Clin Immunol Pract 2016;4(1):38-59; with permission.

None of the Category C criteria are specific but in combination support the diagnosis of probable CVID. Most of the patients with CVID have a reduction of IgA and/or IgM.[1,3] Most are likely to have impaired vaccine responses. We believed it was important to compare antibody responses to those of normal persons, because most patients with CVID who have received their primary immunization series are likely to have generated memory B-cell responses and would be expected to produce protective antibody levels. We were concerned that protective antibody levels as eligibility criteria for SCIG/IVIG were too stringent and would deprive a significant proportion of symptomatic patients who would benefit from such treatment.

Vaccine antibody responses in normal persons have been published.[29–31] Patients receiving a single booster dose of tetanus or diphtheria toxoid should achieve an antibody response of at least 1 IU/mL,[29] although we and other investigators have shown diphtheria toxoid is less immunogenic.[29,32] Adults and children receiving the *Haemophilus influenzae* type B (HIB) vaccine should reach antibody levels of at least 1.0 μg/mL rather than the protective level of 0.15 μg/mL.[30,31]

Although somewhat controversial,[33] we accepted the recommendation of the American Academy of Asthma Allergy and Immunology, which stated that adults receiving the Pneumovax 23 should achieve a protective level of 1.3 μg/mL (or a 2-fold increase) for at least 70% of serotypes, whereas children should reach

---

Box 5
Difficulties undertaking and interpreting vaccine responses in common variable immunodeficiency disorders

Tetanus toxoid
    Excellent immunogen: normal response in severe hypogammaglobulinemia[32]
    Presence of memory B cells from childhood tetanus vaccination can make responses difficult to interpret in patients with CVID[21]
    Results should be compared with normal individuals[29]
    Uncertain validity of using simple antigens with adjuvant to gauge response to pathogens in vivo[20]
    Patients with THI can have impaired tetanus responses[47]

Diphtheria toxoid
    Poor immunogen: responses impaired even in healthy individuals[24,32]
    Presence of memory B cells from childhood diphtheria vaccination can make responses difficult to interpret in patients with CVID[21]
    Response should be compared with normal individuals[29]
    Questionable validity of using simple antigens to gauge response to complex pathogens in vivo[20]
    Patients with THI can have impaired diphtheria responses[47]

Haemophilus influenzae type B (HIB)
    Outstanding immunogen: normal response in symptomatic profoundly hypogammmaglobulinemic patients[32]
    There are major differences in antibody titers between cohorts who have not been immunized versus those who have had HIB as part of their routine vaccines.[58]
    Cannot be used to assess CHO responses as it is conjugated to protein
    Protective levels may not be logical: need to compare with normal persons[30,31]
    Patients with THI can have impaired HIB responses.[47]

Pneumococcal vaccines
    Poor response in asymptomatic, mildly hypogammaglobulinemic patients[32]
    Poor response to PPV in infants younger than 2 years[50]
    Yet up to 18% of patients with CVID respond to PPV[59]
    Differences in responses between middle-aged and elderly adults[60]
    Risk of unresponsiveness with repeated doses of PPV[61]
    Difficulties in measuring antibody responses: assays not standardized[7]
    No commercial assay kits for individual serotypes
    Setting up the serotype assay is technically challenging for diagnostic laboratories.
    Pooled serotype assays less helpful in patients who have received Prevnar 13
    Cross-reactive carbohydrates can interfere with the assay
    Some serotypes (serotype 3) are more immunogenic than others (6B & 23F)[50]
    Different platforms for pneumococcal antibodies may not be comparable[62]
    Use of Prevnar13 as part of routine vaccines will make it difficult to measure responses to carbohydrates
    Mucosal protection may require higher antibody levels than that required to protect against sepsis[63]
    Opsonophagocytic capability of pneumococcal antibodies is important for protection and cannot be easily measured[64]
    Disagreement about protective antibody levels[65–67]
    Diagnostic criteria for a normal response are controversial: at least 5 different criteria in the literature.[33–35]
    Vaccine quality varies: lot to lot variation in stability of conjugated vaccines[50]

Neoantigens
    Not widely used yet, for example, typhoid vaccine[50]
    Many patients with CVID may respond, for example, meningococcal vaccine[68]
    Experimental vaccines not approved by Food and Drug Adminstration φx174[69]
    Risk of adverse reactions to rabies vaccines (in this context)[50]
    Tick-borne encephalitis vaccine not widely available

PPV is administered to test response to T-cell independent carbohydrate antigens, whereas conjugated vaccines such as HIB and toxoids to test responses to T-cell–dependent antigens. *Abbreviation:* PPV, pneumococcal polysaccharide vaccine.

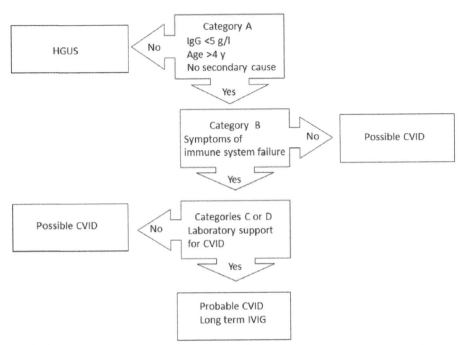

Fig. 1. Treatment algorithm for CVID. Patients must meet all major criteria in Category A for consideration of CVID. Category B confirms the presence of symptoms indicating ISF. To have probable CVID, patients must also have supportive laboratory evidence of immune system dysfunction (Category C) or characteristic histologic lesions of CVID (Category D). Patients with mild hypogammaglobulinemia (IgG >5 g/L) are termed hypogammaglobulinemia of uncertain significance (HGUS). Symptomatic patients are designated sHGUS and those without symptoms are designated aHGUS. Patients meeting Category A criteria but not other criteria are deemed to have possible CVID. Most patients with probable CVID are likely to require IVG/SCIG. Some patients with possible CVID will require IVIG/SCIG but most patients with HGUS are unlikely to need IVIG/SCIG replacement. (*From* Ameratunga R, Woon ST, Gillis D, et al. New diagnostic criteria for common variable immune deficiency (CVID), which may assist with decisions to treat with intravenous or subcutaneous immunoglobulin. Clin Exp Immunol 2013;174(2):208; with permission.)

50%.[34,35] Adequate but transient vaccine responses are also included in Category C of the Ameratunga and colleagues[21] (2013) criteria, which may reflect in vivo failure of B-cell memory responses in some patients.[36]

Although absent isohemagglutinins are part of The Ameratunga and colleagues (2013) and ESID/PAGID (1999) criteria, in our experience it is rare for a diagnosis of CVID to be made purely based on absent isohemagglutinins in a patient with reduced IgG and IgA (or IgM) levels.

Most patients with CVID have reduced memory B cells, and these constitute a diagnostic criterion in Category C.[8] It is however important for memory B-cell subsets to be measured on at least 2 occasions, as we have shown the numbers can vary on repeat testing.[37] Genetic predisposition to CVID including mutations of TACI (*TNFRSF13B*), BAFFR (*TNFRSF13C*), TWEAK (*TNFSF12*), *MSH5*, and TRAIL (*TNFSF10*) is included in our Category C diagnostic criteria.

Disproportionate reduction or deficiency of IgG3 was included in our criteria, as there is peer-reviewed literature suggesting IgG3 deficiency should be considered an important biomarker for a humoral immune defect.[38,39] We have included serologic manifestations of significant autoimmunity in Category C, which would include positive tests for lupus anticoagulant, Coombes test etc. In most large series of patients with CVID there are approximately 15% to 25% of patients who have severe autoimmunity and some have minimal infections in spite of their profound hypogammaglobulinemia.

Finally, some patients with CVID have characteristic histologic findings, which have been included in the Ameratunga and colleagues (2013) criteria (Category D). Most of the histologic lesions described in Category D can occur in other disorders. Because Category D will only apply if patients have already met Category A and B criteria (see **Fig. 1**), this will confer specificity for CVID. We have shown on several occasions, that careful review of Category C and D criteria may help identify secondary causes of hypogammaglobulinemia.[40–44]

The Revised ESID Registry (2014) Criteria for Common Variable Immunodeficiency Disorders

The revised ESID registry (2014) criteria for probable CVID were subsequently published in 2014 (see **Box 3**) and are similar to the Ameratunga and colleagues (2013) criteria. In contrast to the previous ESID/PAGID (1999) criteria, patients are required to have symptoms from their immune deficiency or in the case of asymptomatic individuals, a family history of antibody deficiency, to be eligible for a diagnosis of probable CVID. Increased susceptibility to infections along with autoimmunity, unexplained polyclonal lymphoproliferation, or granulomatous disease qualifies patients for further consideration of CVID.

Patients are required to have a "marked decrease" of IgG as well as IgA with or without a reduction in IgM. Again, this is defined as Ig levels 2 SD less than mean for the relevant age appropriate population. Ig levels need to be repeated to confirm persistent reduction. This would exclude transient reductions in Igs that can occur following viral infections or medications.[45] Patients with hypogammaglobulinemia must then have either impaired antibody responses to vaccines, absent isohemagglutinins, or reduced numbers of switched memory B cells for further consideration of probable CVID (see **Box 3**).

The revised ESID registry (2014) criteria have set the vaccine challenge threshold at failure to reach protective levels, rather than the higher community-based thresholds in the Ameratunga and colleagues (2013) criteria. As the Ameratunga and colleagues (2013) criteria, it is possible for patients to qualify as having CVID with normal vaccine challenge responses if they either have absent isohemagglutinins or reduced switched memory B cells less than 70% of the normal population (see **Box 3**). As the Ameratunga and colleagues (2013) criteria, reduced memory B cells in the revised ESID registry (2014) criteria are not mandatory and patients may still qualify for the diagnosis if they have impaired vaccine responses or absent isohemagglutinins.

Granulomatous disease and lymphoproliferation are included in the initial set of clinical criteria in the revised ESID registry (2014) criteria (see **Box 3**). Although not explicitly stated, our interpretation is that lymphoproliferation will include nodular lymphoid hyperplasia of the gut, nodular regenerative hyperplasia of the liver, and GLILD. This will require histologic confirmation or characteristic radiological features in the case of GLILD. Absence of plasma cells in biopsies is however not included in the revised ESID (2014) criteria.

In contrast to the Ameratunga and colleagues (2013) criteria, transient vaccine responses, sequence variations in genes predisposing to CVID, or IgG3 deficiency are not included in the revised ESID registry (2014) criteria.

The Common Variable Immunodeficiency Disorders International Consensus Criteria (2016)

In 2016, a group of immunologists published the ICON for definite CVID (see **Box 4**).[46] Patients were required to have a marked reduction in IgG, again 2 SD less than mean, as well as a decrease in IgM or IgA. In contrast to the revised ESID registry (2014) criteria, reduction of IgA was not mandatory for the ICON (2016) criteria. As the revised ESID registry (2014) criteria, the IgG level had to be repeated in the ICON (2016) criteria.

The ICON (2016) criteria were very similar to the original ESID/PAGID (1999) criteria, as impaired vaccine responses were pivotal in the diagnosis of CVID. Unlike other criteria, which allow a probable or possible diagnosis, the ICON (2016) criteria claimed to be able to make a definite diagnosis of CVID based on a single abnormal vaccine response, which failed to reach protective levels. As with other criteria, the number and types of vaccines were not specified.

The ICON (2016) criteria did not include the characteristic histologic features, reduced memory B cells, IgG subclass deficiency, absent isohemagglutinins, or variants in genes predisposing to CVID. Similarly, no reference was made to poor durability of vaccine responses.

As with all criteria described here, secondary causes of hypogammaglobulinemia had to be excluded. The previous ESID/PAGID (1999) criteria specified 2 years as the eligible age for diagnosis, whereas the Ameratunga and colleagues (2013) criteria, revised ESID registry (2014), and ICON (2016) criteria have raised the age of diagnosis to 4 years. The older age for diagnosis would help exclude monogenic B-cell defects as well as many (but not all) cases of transient hypogammaglobulinemia of infancy (THI).[47] Unlike the ESID/PAGID (1999) and Ameratunga and colleagues (2013) criteria, the revised ESID registry (2014) and ICON (2016) criteria exclude severe T-cell defects from the spectrum of CVID, because these patients are deemed to have an LOCID.

STUDIES THAT HAVE COMPARED THESE CRITERIA

We are aware of 3 studies to date, which have compared these criteria in the same group of patients. Selenius and colleagues[48] compared the performance of the ESID/PAGID (1999), the Ameratunga and colleagues (2013), and the ICON (2016) criteria in their patients from Finland. In their study, the ESID/PAGID (1999) criteria and the Ameratunga and colleagues (2013) criteria performed similarly. In contrast, the ICON (2016) criteria identified far fewer patients, mainly because of the lack of vaccine response studies in many of these patients, who had been on long-term IVIG. Selenius and colleagues did not believe the revised ESID registry (2014) criteria were useful because of the requirement for mandatory reduction of IgA as well as IgG to establish the diagnosis.

In another recent study from Denmark, all patients with CVID were identified from ICD codes from the national patient registry.[49] In this study, 179 patients were identified with CVID, of whom 95% were on SCIG/IVIG. Many had not had detailed immunologic studies before commencing treatment. Application of the Ameratunga and colleagues (2013) criteria showed 24 (13.4%) patients had "probable CVID," 106 (59.2%) patients had "possible CVID," and 49 (27.4%) patients were categorized as "inadequate investigation". This study also used the previous PAGID/ESID (1999) criteria but not the revised ESID (2014) registry or ICON (2016) criteria. According to the ESID/PAGID (1999) criteria, 50 (27.9%) patients were categorized as "probable CVID," 6 (3.4%) patients were categorized as "possible CVID," and 123 (68.7%) patients could not be categorized due to inadequate investigation. It would seem the Ameratunga and colleagues (2013) criteria performed better in these 2 studies, where patients were mostly on SCIG/IVIG.

We have recently published the results from the New Zealand hypogammaglobulinemia study (NZHS), which began in 2006.[32] This long-term prospective cohort study examined the natural history of patients with hypogammaglobulinemia who were not immediately commenced on SCIG/IVIG. This study has shown that many asymptomatic patients with profound (IgG <3 g/L) hypogammaglobulinemia who declined SCIG/IVIG and those with moderate (IgG 3–6.9 g/L) hypogammaglobulinemia have remained well for over a decade. In contrast, patients with symptomatic hypogammaglobulinemia were much more likely to be offered SCIG/IVIG.

Unexpectedly, the NZHS also showed 41.6% (20/48) of symptomatic patients normalized their IgG on at least one occasion. Seven of twelve hypogammaglobulinemic patients with bronchiectasis were also able to spontaneously normalize their IgG on at least one occasion.[32] We have termed this phenomenon transient hypogammaglobulinemia of adulthood (THA). Only one asymptomatic (out of 55) and 2 symptomatic (out of 48) patients with THA increased their IgG from less than 5 g/L to the normal range. THA has important implications for CVID diagnostic criteria with an IgG threshold of 7 g/L. Either the threshold for IgG will have to be substantially lowered or IgG levels will need to be monitored for much longer periods before a probable or definite diagnosis of CVID can be made.

The other important finding from this study was that vaccine challenge responses did not discriminate between those who were offered SCIG/IVIG from those who have remained well for extended periods. We showed that Pneumovax 23 and diphtheria antibody responses were equally impaired in asymptomatic healthy individuals with mild hypogammaglobulinemia compared with those with severe symptomatic hypogammaglobulinemia, including patients who were offered SCIG/IVIG. In contrast, the tetanus and HIB vaccines produced outstanding responses in the asymptomatic group as well those with severe symptomatic hypogammaglobulinemia, including mostly who were accepted for SCIG/IVIG. In the NZHS, commonly used vaccines were thus nondiscriminatory and in our view, adds uncertainty to the value of vaccine studies in CVID (see **Box 5**). It is possible neoantigens may have discriminated between these groups of patients more accurately. There are, however, barriers to their routine use at this time. Most neoantigens are not always easily accessible and there are safety concerns about the rabies vaccine in this context.[50]

We compared the utility of CVID diagnostic criteria in the NZHS. The Ameratunga and colleagues (2013) and the revised ESID registry (2014) criteria identified a similar group of patients although there were differences because of the requirement for symptoms in the Ameratunga and colleagues (2013) criteria. We could not directly compare the performance of the ICON (2016) criteria, as these require impaired vaccine responses, which are discretionary in the Ameratunga and colleagues (2013) and revised ESID registry (2014) criteria. There would thus be a risk of circular logic if the diagnostic performance of all 3 criteria is compared, based on impaired vaccine responses. In our study, many healthy asymptomatic patients with mild hypogammaglobulinemia who had impaired vaccine responses have remained well for a mean duration approaching a decade. It seems unlikely these patients have definite CVID or any other immunologic disorder.

APPLICATION OF THESE COMMON VARIABLE IMMUNODEFICIENCY DISORDERS DIAGNOSTIC CRITERIA TO SPECIFIC CLINICAL SCENARIOS
Asymptomatic Individuals

There is debate about whether symptoms are a mandatory requirement for diagnosing CVID. The original ESID/PAGID (1999) CVID diagnostic criteria did not specify requirement for symptoms.[22] Thus, as noted earlier, asymptomatic patients with trivial reductions in IgG and IgA levels with impaired diphtheria vaccine responses could be diagnosed with probable CVID and offered life-long SCIG/IVIG. The revised ESID registry criteria (2014) allow asymptomatic patients to be diagnosed as having CVID if they have a relative with immunodeficiency. The ICON criteria also allow asymptomatic patients to be diagnosed with definitive CVID, provided Category 2 to 5 criteria are met (see **Box 4**).

Our criteria, in contrast, do not allow asymptomatic individuals to be diagnosed with probable CVID, as they do not meet the Category B criteria, which are clinical sequelae of the disorder. The only exception is the coincidental discovery of an asymptomatic characteristic CVID lesion such as GLILD, during the course of unrelated investigations in a patient subsequently shown to have primary hypogammaglobulinemia.[32] None of the asymptomatic patients in the NZHS developed bronchiectasis over the mean follow-up period of 106 months. Given the marked differences in prognosis in the NZHS, in our view, clinical sequelae should be a mandatory component of CVID diagnostic criteria. Symptoms seem to be a better prognostic indicator than laboratory tests, especially given the difficulties with vaccine challenge responses (see **Box 5**).

Subcutaneous Immunoglobulin/Intravenous Immunoglobulin Treatment in Patients Not Meeting Common Variable Immunodeficiency Disorders Diagnostic Criteria

There are many patients with primary hypogammaglobulinemia who do not meet criteria for CVID. The previous ESID/PAGID (1999) criteria had a category of possible CVID for patients not meeting the complete criteria for CVID (see **Box 1**). The revised ESID registry (2014) criteria have a category of unclassified hypogammaglobulinemia (UCH) for patients who do not meet all the criteria for CVID. Hypogammaglobulinemic patients not meeting the ICON criteria are deemed to have unspecified hypogammaglobulinemia (USH). No recommendations have been made about eligibility for SCIG/IVIG for patients within these 3 criteria. Other investigators have designated such patients as idiopathic primary hypogammaglobulinemic (IPH) or IgG deficient (IgGD).[51,52] It is common for patients with IPH, UCH, IgGD, or USH to be accepted for SCIG/IVIG treatment even though they do not meet criteria for CVID.

We have designated a category of possible CVID for those patients meeting Category A criteria (or AC or AD) but not Category B criteria (see **Fig. 1**). We have stated such asymptomatic patients with profound hypogammaglobulinemia should be treated with SCIG/IVIG, as they may be at risk of severe bacterial infections.[20]

There are other patients who have mild hypogammaglobulinemia (IgG > 5 g/L) who are otherwise well or who have symptoms of varying severity. These patients are termed hypogammaglobulinemia of uncertain significance (HGUS).[21] We have shown it is useful to subclassify HGUS patients depending on whether (sHGUS) or not (aHGUS) they have symptoms attributable to immune system failure.[32] The NZHS has shown that only one asymptomatic patient (of 59) in our study experienced progressive decline in IgG levels needing IVIG.[32] We have stated some patients with sHGUS with bronchiectasis, for example, may need to be treated with SCIG/IVIG, provided they do not have THA (see **Fig. 1**), regardless of vaccine responses.

Diagnosis of Common Variable Immunodeficiency Disorders in Patients Already Treated with Subcutaneous Immunoglobulin/Intravenous Immunoglobulin or on Immunosuppression

It is difficult to assess standard laboratory criteria for CVID if a patient is being treated with SCIG/IVIG or is on immunosuppression for autoimmunity. Diagnostic criteria based primarily on conventional vaccine responses (ESID/PAGID 1999 and ICON 2016) cannot be applied in this situation. This was illustrated in the Danish national CVID study, where many had not had vaccine challenge responses before starting treatment.[49]

There is now a strong argument for undertaking routine genetic sequencing in all patients with a CVID phenotype, if resources permit.[53] If a causative mutation is identified, symptomatic patients with hypogammaglobulinemia should be placed on long-term SCIG/IVIG. CVID diagnostic criteria are no longer relevant in this situation, as the patient would be deemed to have a PID/IEI caused by a specific mutation.

Similarly, incorporating histologic features in the diagnostic criteria may be useful where patients have already commenced SCIG/IVIG, as there are risks in stopping treatment to undertake other investigations.[21,54] We were recently able to identify sarcoidosis and exclude CVID in a patient with hypogammaglobulinemia, who was on long-term immunosuppression for severe autoimmunity.[44] This patient's lymph nodes showed the presence of granulomas and plasma cells with intact germinal centers, which made the granulomatous variant of CVID (GVCVID) very unlikely. Subsequently when immunosuppression was lifted, his IgG normalized, confirming he did not have GVCVID.

We have recently identified another patient with THI who was treated for more than a decade with IVIG before the diagnosis was made at age 32 years.[47] His IgG normalized after stopping IVIG. In his case, the normal IgA and IgM levels coupled with normal memory B cells were important clues this patient did not have CVID. Both the Ameratunga and colleagues (2013) and the revised ESID registry (2014) criteria were useful in excluding CVID in this patient.

Retrospective Diagnosis of Common Variable Immunodeficiency Disorders in Deceased Patients

It can be difficult to retrospectively determine if a patient had CVID if they are deceased. Histology can be very helpful in this situation. If a patient with primary hypogammaglobulinemia is found to have had any of the characteristic histologic findings before death or at autopsy, a retrospective diagnosis of CVID could be made using the Ameratunga and colleagues (2013) criteria.

It may be possible to identify patients with CVID-like disorders using archived specimens. Tissue blocks and Guthrie cards can be retrieved and sequenced for causative genes following death. This could potentially identify a CVID-like disorder in a deceased patient.

Malignancy

Patients with CVID and CVID-like disorders have an increased risk of malignancy. The Ameratunga and colleagues (2013), the revised ESID (2014) registry, and ICON (2016) criteria do not attempt to address the complex situation of hypogammaglobulinemia/CVID associated with malignancy. It can be very difficult to determine if hypogammaglobulinemia/CVID is the cause or the result of treating the malignancy. In the presence of malignancy, genetic testing can be helpful. If a patient with malignancy has a causative mutation (*NFKB1, NFKB2* etc.), they can be reclassified as having a CVID-like disorder.

SUMMARY

Current diagnostic criteria reflect the evolution in the understanding of CVID. We do not believe a definitive diagnosis of CVID can be made until the molecular basis of this group of disorders is identified. In nonconsanguineous populations, the genetic basis for most patients with a CVID phenotype is currently unknown. There may be future technological innovations analogous to the current NGS revolution, which may allow elucidation of the molecular basis of all remaining patients with a diagnosis of CVID. Counterintuitively, the disorders we currently term CVID will cease to exist once every patient has a clear genetic diagnosis.[15]

ACKNOWLEDGMENTS

The authors thank our patients for participating in these studies for the benefit of others. In turn, we hope our analysis of various CVID diagnostic and treatment criteria will assist our patients, colleagues, and funders of SCIG/IVIG. The authors thank the AMRF, A + Trust, and IDFNZ for grant support. The authors thank colleagues from around the world for their valuable comments.

COMPETING INTERESTS

The authors declare they have no competing interests.

REFERENCES

1. Cunningham-Rundles C, Bodian C. Common variable immunodeficiency: clinical and immunological features of 248 patients. Clin Immunol 1999;92(1):34–48.
2. Quinti I, Soresina A, Spadaro G, et al. Long-term follow-up and outcome of a large cohort of patients with common variable immunodeficiency. J Clin Immunol 2007;27(3):308–16.
3. Chapel H, Lucas M, Lee M, et al. Common variable immunodeficiency disorders: division into distinct clinical phenotypes. Blood 2008;112(2):277–86.
4. Ameratunga R. Assessing disease severity in Common Variable Immunodeficiency Disorders (CVID) and CVID-like disorders. Front Immunol 2018;9:2130.
5. Gathmann B, Mahlaoui N2, CEREDIH, et al. Clinical picture and treatment of 2212 patients with common variable immunodeficiency. J Allergy Clin Immunol 2014; 134(1):116–26.
6. Oksenhendler E, Gérard L, Fieschi C, et al. Infections in 252 patients with common variable immunodeficiency. Clin Infect Dis 2008;46(10):1547–54.
7. Ballow M. Vaccines in the assessment of patients for immune deficiency. J Allergy Clin Immunol 2012;130(1):283–4.e5.
8. Wehr C, Kivioja T, Schmitt C, et al. The EUROclass trial: defining subgroups in common variable immunodeficiency. Blood 2008;111(1):77–85.
9. Malphettes M, Gérard L, Carmagnat M, et al. Late-onset combined immune deficiency: a subset of common variable immunodeficiency with severe T cell defect. Clin Infect Dis 2009;49(9):1329–38.

10. Ameratunga R, Ahn Y, Jordan A, et al. Keeping it in the family: the case for considering late onset combined immunodeficiency a subset of common variable immunodeficiency disorders. Expert Rev Clin Immunol 2018;14(7):549–56.

11. Ameratunga R, Becroft DM, Hunter W. The simultaneous presentation of sarcoidosis and common variable immune deficiency. Pathology 2000;32(4):280–2.

12. Fasano MB, Sullivan KE, Sarpong SB, et al. Sarcoidosis and common variable immunodeficiency.Report of 8 cases and review of the literature. Medicine (Baltimore) 1996;75(5):251–61.

13. Malamut G, Verkarre V, Suarez F, et al. The enteropathy associated with common variable immunodeficiency: the delineated frontiers with celiac disease. Am J Gastroenterol 2010;105(10):2262–75.

14. Abolhassani H, Hammarstrom L, Cunningham-Rundles C. Current genetic landscape in common variable immune deficiency. Blood 2020;15(431026): 2019000929.

15. Ameratunga R, Lehnert K, Woon ST, et al. Review: diagnosing common variable immunodeficiency disorder in the era of genome sequencing. Clin Rev Allergy Immunol 2018;54(2):261–8.

16. Maffucci P, Filion CA, Boisson B, et al. Genetic diagnosis using whole exome sequencing in common variable immunodeficiency. Front Immunol 2016;7:220.

17. Ameratunga R, Koopmans W1, Woon ST1, et al. Epistatic interactions between mutations of TACI (TNFRSF13B) and TCF3 result in a severe primary immunodeficiency disorder and systemic lupus erythematosus. Clin Transl Immunol 2017; 6(10):e159.

18. Ameratunga R, Woon ST, Bryant VL, et al. Clinical implications of digenic inheritiance and epistasis in primary immunodeficiency disorders. Front Immunol 2018; 8:1965.

19. Pan-Hammarstrom Q, Salzer U, Du L, et al. Reexamining the role of TACI coding variants in common variable immunodeficiency and selective IgA deficiency. Nat Genet 2007;39(4):429–30.

20. Koopmans W, Woon ST, Brooks AE, et al. Clinical variability of family members with the C104R mutation in transmembrane activator and calcium modulator and cyclophilin ligand interactor (TACI). J Clin Immunol 2013;33(1):68–73.

21. Ameratunga R, Woon ST, Gillis D, et al. New diagnostic criteria for common variable immune deficiency (CVID), which may assist with decisions to treat with intravenous or subcutaneous immunoglobulin. Clin Exp Immunol 2013;174(2): 203–11.

22. Conley ME, Notarangelo LD, Etzioni A. Diagnostic criteria for primary immunodeficiencies.Representing PAGID (Pan-American Group for Immunodeficiency) and ESID (European Society for Immunodeficiencies). Clin Immunol 1999;93(3): 190–7.

23. Ritchie RF, Palomaki GE, Neveux LM, et al. Reference distributions for immunoglobulins A, G, and M: a practical, simple, and clinically relevant approach in a large cohort. J Clin Lab Anal 1998;12(6):363–70.

24. Chapel H, Cunningham-Rundles C. Update in understanding common variable immunodeficiency disorders (CVIDs) and the management of patients with these conditions. Br J Haematol 2009;145(6):709–27.

25. Seppanen M, Aghamohammadi A, Rezaei N. Is there a need to redefine the diagnostic criteria for common variable immunodeficiency? Expert Rev Clin Immunol 2014;10(1):1–5.

26. Yong PF, Thaventhiran JE, Grimbacher B. "A rose is a rose is a rose," but CVID is Not CVID common variable immune deficiency (CVID), what do we know in 2011? Adv Immunol 2011;111:47–107.

27. Ameratunga R, Storey P, Barker R, et al. Application of diagnostic and treatment criteria for common variable immunodeficiency disorder. Expert Rev Clin Immunol 2015;12(3):257–66.

28. Ameratunga R, Woon ST, Gillis D, et al. New diagnostic criteria for CVID. Expert Rev Clin Immunol 2014;10(2):183–6.

29. Thierry-Carstensen B, Jordan K, Uhlving HH, et al. A randomised, double-blind, non-inferiority clinical trial on the safety and immunogenicity of a tetanus, diphtheria and monocomponent acellular pertussis (TdaP) vaccine in comparison to a tetanus and diphtheria (Td) vaccine when given as booster vaccinations to healthy adults. Vaccine 2012;30(37):5464–71.

30. Hawdon N, Nix EB, Tsang RS, et al. Immune response to Haemophilus influenzae type b vaccination in patients with chronic renal failure. Clin Vaccine Immunol 2012;19(6):967–9.

31. Dentinger CM, Hennessy TW, Bulkow LR, et al. Immunogenicity and reactogenicity to Haemophilus influenzae type B (Hib) conjugate vaccine among rural Alaska adults. Hum Vaccin 2006;2(1):24–8.

32. Ameratunga R, Ahn Y, Steele R, et al. The natural history of untreated primary hypogammaglobulinemia in adults: implications for the diagnosis and treatment of Common Variable Immunodeficiency Disorders (CVID). Front Immunol 2019; 17(10):1541.

33. Beck SC. Making sense of serotype-specific pneumococcal antibody measurements. Ann Clin Biochem 2013;50(Pt 6):517–9.

34. Bonilla FA, Bernstein IL, Khan DA, et al. Practice parameter for the diagnosis and management of primary immunodeficiency. Ann AllergyAsthma Immunol 2005; 94(5 Suppl 1):S1–63.

35. Paris K, Sorensen RU. Assessment and clinical interpretation of polysaccharide antibody responses. Ann AllergyAsthma Immunol 2007;99(5):462–4.

36. Grabenstein JD, Manoff SB. Pneumococcal polysaccharide 23-valent vaccine: long-term persistence of circulating antibody and immunogenicity and safety after revaccination in adults. Vaccine 2012;30(30):4435–44.

37. Koopmans W, Woon ST, Zeng IS, et al. Variability of memory B cell markers in a cohort of Common Variable Immune Deficiency patients over six months. Scand J Immunol 2013;77(6):470–5.

38. Abrahamian F, Agrawal S, Gupta S. Immunological and clinical profile of adult patients with selective immunoglobulin subclass deficiency: response to intravenous immunoglobulin therapy. Clin Exp Immunol 2010;159(3):344–50.

39. Olinder-Nielsen AM, Granert C, Forsberg P, et al. Immunoglobulin prophylaxis in 350 adults with IgG subclass deficiency and recurrent respiratory tract infections: a long-term follow-up. Scand J Infect Dis 2007;39(1):44–50.

40. Ameratunga RV, Casey P, Parry S, et al. Hypogammaglobulinemia factitia. Munchausen syndrome presenting as Common Variable Immune Deficiency. Allergy Asthma Clin Immunol 2013;9:36.

41. Empson M, Sinclair J, O'Donnell J, et al. The assessment and management of primary antibody deficiency. N Z Med J 2004;117(1195):U914.

42. Ameratunga R, Barker RW, Steele RH, et al. Profound reversible hypogammaglobulinemia caused by celiac disease in the absence of protein losing enteropathy. J Clin Immunol 2015;35(6):589–94.

43. Ameratunga R, Lindsay K, Woon, S-T, et al. New diagnostic criteria could distinguish common variable immunodeficiency disorder from anticonvulsant-induced hypogammaglobulinemia. Clin Exp Neuroimmunol 2015;6(1):83–8.
44. Ameratunga R, Ahn Y, Tse D, et al. The critical role of histology in distinguishing sarcoidosis from common variable immunodeficiency disorder (CVID) in a patient with hypogammaglobulinemia. AllergyAsthma Clin Immunol 2019;15:78.
45. Smith J, Fernando T, McGrath N, et al. Lamotrigine-induced common variable immune deficiency. Neurology 2004;62(5):833–4.
46. Bonilla FA, Barlan I, Chapel H, et al. International Consensus Document (ICON): common variable immunodeficiency disorders. J Allergy Clin Immunol Pract 2016;4(1):38–59.
47. Ameratunga R, Ahn Y, Steele R, et al. Transient hypogammaglobulinemia of infancy: many patients recover in adolescence and adulthood. Clin Exp Immunol 2019;198(2):224–32.
48. Selenius JS, Martelius T, Pikkarainen S, et al. Unexpectedly high prevalence of common variable immunodeficiency in Finland. Front Immunol 2017;8:1190.
49. Westh L, Mogensen TH, Dalgaard LS, et al. Identification and characterization of a nationwide danish adult common variable immunodeficiency cohort. Scand J Immunol 2017;85(6):450–61.
50. Orange JS, Ballow M, Stiehm ER, et al. Use and interpretation of diagnostic vaccination in primary immunodeficiency: a working group report of the Basic and Clinical Immunology Interest Section of the American Academy of Allergy, Asthma & Immunology. J Allergy Clin Immunol 2012;130(3 Suppl):S1–24.
51. Driessen GJ, Dalm VA, van Hagen PM, et al. Common variable immunodeficiency and idiopathic primary hypogammaglobulinemia: two different conditions within the same disease spectrum. Haematologica 2013;98(10):1617–23.
52. Filion CA, Taylor-Black S, Maglione PJ, et al. Differentiation of common variable immunodeficiency from IgG deficiency. J Allergy Clin Immunol Pract 2019;7(4):1277–84.
53. Ameratunga R, Woon ST. Perspective: evolving concepts in the diagnosis and understanding of Common Variable Immunodeficiency Disorders (CVID). Clin Rev Allergy Immunol 2019. [Epub ahead of print]. https://doi.org/10.1007/s12016-019-08765-6.
54. Daniels JA, Gibson MK, Xu L, et al. Gastrointestinal tract pathology in patients with common variable immunodeficiency (CVID): a clinicopathologic study and review. Am J Surg Pathol 2007;31(12):1800–12.
55. Musher DM, Manof SB, Liss C, et al. Safety and antibody response, including antibody persistence for 5 years, after primary vaccination or revaccination with pneumococcal polysaccharide vaccine in middle-aged and older adults. J Infect Dis 2010;201(4):516–24.
56. Fuss IJ, Friend J, Yang Z, et al. Nodular regenerative hyperplasia in common variable immunodeficiency. J Clin Immunol 2013;33(4):748–58.
57. Malamut G, Ziol M, Suarez F, et al. Nodular regenerative hyperplasia: the main liver disease in patients with primary hypogammaglobulinemia and hepatic abnormalities. J Hepatol 2008;48(1):74–82.
58. Ladhani S, Ramsay M, Flood J, et al. Haemophilus influenzae serotype B (Hib) seroprevalence in England and Wales in 2009. Euro Surveill 2012;17:46.
59. Goldacker S, Draeger R, Warnatz K, et al. Active vaccination in patients with common variable immunodeficiency (CVID). Clin Immunol 2007;124(3):294–303.
60. Lee H, Nahm MH, Kim KH. The effect of age on the response to the pneumococcal polysaccharide vaccine. BMC Infect Dis 2010;10:60.

61. O'Brien KL, Hochman M, Goldblatt D. Combined schedules of pneumococcal conjugate and polysaccharide vaccines: is hyporesponsiveness an issue? Lancet Infect Dis 2007;7(9):597–606.
62. Balloch A, Licciardi PV, Tang ML. Serotype-specific anti-pneumococcal IgG and immune competence: critical differences in interpretation criteria when different methods are used. J Clin Immunol 2013;33(2):335–41.
63. Jokinen JT, Ahman H, Kilpi TM, et al. Concentration of antipneumococcal antibodies as a serological correlate of protection: an application to acute otitis media. J Infect Dis 2004;190(3):545–50.
64. Russell FM, Carapetis JR, Burton RL, et al. Opsonophagocytic activity following a reduced dose 7-valent pneumococcal conjugate vaccine infant primary series and 23-valent pneumococcal polysaccharide vaccine at 12 months of age. Vaccine 2011;29(3):535–44.
65. Jodar L, Butler J, Carlone G, et al. Serological criteria for evaluation and licensure of new pneumococcal conjugate vaccine formulations for use in infants. Vaccine 2003;21(23):3265–72.
66. Lee LH, Frasch CE, Falk LA, et al. Correlates of immunity for pneumococcal conjugate vaccines. Vaccine 2003;21(17–18):2190–6.
67. Ameratunga R, Woon ST, Neas K, et al. The clinical utility of molecular diagnostic testing for primary immune deficiency disorders: a case based review. AllergyAsthma Clin Immunol 2010;6(1):12.
68. Rezaei N, Siadat SD, Aghamohammadi A, et al. Serum bactericidal antibody response 1 year after meningococcal polysaccharide vaccination of patients with common variable immunodeficiency. Clin Vaccine Immunol 2010;17(4): 524–8.
69. Ochs HD, Davis SD, Wedgwood RJ. Immunologic responses to bacteriophage phi-X 174 in immunodeficiency diseases. J Clin Invest 1971;50(12):2559–68.

Vaccines in Patients with Primary Immune Deficiency

Francisco A. Bonilla, MD, PhD

KEYWORDS

- Vaccines • Primary immunodeficiency • Immunology

KEY POINTS

- Vaccines are of critical importance for the diagnosis and management of primary immune deficiency.
- Knowledge of vaccine composition and function is central to understanding these clinical uses of vaccines.
- IgG therapy has an impact on the diagnostic and clinical use of vaccines in primary immune deficiency.

INTRODUCTION

The goal of vaccination (or immunization) is to prevent disease by the intentional exposure of a host to an infectious agent or to some of its components. Via the induction of immunologic memory, this controlled exposure prevents or mitigates future disease caused by the infectious agent.[1,2] Vaccines are among the earliest interventions undertaken to prevent human infectious disease. The practice of variolation, scraping the skin of healthy people with crusts of smallpox lesions to intentionally cause an infection, was performed 1000 years ago in China.[3] Of course, a wide variety of vaccines are in clinical use today. They represent the single most important medical technology to prevent disease. Billions of deaths worldwide have been avoided since the beginning of the "modern" vaccine era conceptually with Edward Jenner and many others in the late eighteenth and nineteenth centuries, and with more widespread application around the world starting in the mid-twentieth century with polio vaccine.[3] **Table 1** lists vaccines in current use.

Vaccines are broadly categorized into two types: viable and nonviable.[1,2] Viable vaccines are infectious agents (viruses or bacteria) that are capable of causing an infection and replicating in the host. These agents are "attenuated"; they are less virulent variants of wild-type organisms, and they cause milder disease in comparison with the wild-type agents. Nonviable vaccines contain noninfectious killed whole

Northeast Allergy, Asthma & Immunology, 79 Erdman Way, Suite 101, Leominster, MA 01453, USA
E-mail address: fabmd1@verizon.net

Immunol Allergy Clin N Am 40 (2020) 421–435
https://doi.org/10.1016/j.iac.2020.03.004
0889-8561/20/© 2020 Elsevier Inc. All rights reserved.
immunology.theclinics.com

Table 1
Vaccines in routine current use

Antigens(s)	Vaccine Composition	TD or TI	Protective Level	Seroconversion Rate (%)[a]
Inactive or Subunit Vaccines				
Tetanus toxoid	Protein	TD	0.1 IU/mL	100
Acellular pertussis	Protein	TD	NA[b]	NA
Diphtheria toxoid	Protein	TD	0.1 IU/mL	99
Hepatitis A	Inactivated virus	TD	20 mIU/mL	99–100
Hepatitis B	Recombinant protein	TD	>10 mIU/mL	98–99
Haemophilus influenzae type B (HIB) capsular polysaccharide (poly-ribose phosphate [PRP])	Polysaccharide (PS) conjugate	TD	1 µg/mL	80–100
Human papilloma virus	Recombinant protein	TD	NA	NA
Influenza (injection)	Inactivated virus	TD	NA	NA
Meningococcal capsular polysaccharide (types A, C, W, Y)	PS conjugate vaccine (4 valent)	TD	Titer >1:8	50–100[c]
Meningococcal capsular polysaccharide (type B)	PS conjugate vaccine (2 valent)	TD	Titer >1:8	50–100[c]
Pneumococcal capsular polysaccharide	PS conjugate vaccine (PCV), Prevnar 13 (13 valent)	TD	0.35 µg/mL	64–98[c]
Pneumococcal capsular polysaccharide	Pure PS vaccine (PPSV), PNEUMOVAX 23 (23 valent)	TI	1.3 µg/mL	2-fold increase, 25–100; 4-fold, 0–100[c]
Polio virus	Inactivated virus	TD	Titer >1:4	95–100 after 2 doses
Live Agent Vaccines				
Influenza (nasal)	Attenuated virus	TD	NA	NA
Measles	Attenuated virus	TD	>1.1 EIU/mL	1 dose, 95–99; 2 doses, 100
Mumps	Attenuated virus	TD	>1.1 EIU/mL	1 dose, 95–99; 2 doses, 100

(continued on next page)

Table 1 (continued)				
Antigens(s)	Vaccine Composition	TD or TI	Protective Level	Seroconversion Rate (%)[a]
Rotavirus	Reassortment attenuated virus	TD	Rotavirus IgA >20 U/mL	77–87
Rubella	Attenuated virus	TD	>1.1 EIU/mL	1 dose, 95–99; 2 doses, 100
Varicella	Attenuated virus	TD	5 glycoprotein-ELISA U/mL	1 dose, 85; 2 doses, 100
Bacille Calmette-Guerin	Attenuated mycobacterium	TD	NA	NA

[a] This information can be found in the prescribing information summary for each vaccine. They are available on all of the vaccine manufacturers' websites, as well as many other internet resources including the Immunization Action Coalition (http://www.immunize.org).
[b] NA, not applicable. The protective level is undefined or the antigen(s) are not used for immune deficiency diagnosis or therapeutic monitoring.
[c] Varies widely with serotype, age, and study.

organisms or subcomponents of the organism. Both types of vaccines are capable of generating robust humoral immune responses that form the basis of protection from future exposure. Attenuated live vaccine organisms are also capable of generating effective cellular immunity, whereas nonviable vaccines usually do so only weakly, if at all.

With respect to the induction of a humoral immune response, the antigenic components of microbes (and other immunogens) are often categorized as T-dependent (TD) or T-independent (TI).[4] Protein and glycoprotein antigens are TD and B cells require help from T cells to become fully activated and generate antibody-forming cells (plasma cells). TI antigens are macromolecules with repeating identical subunits, such as complex polysaccharides that are capable of cross-linking immunoglobulin on B cells and activating accessory dendritic or mononuclear cells to produce cytokines that can drive development of plasma cells without participation of T cells. Most of the vaccines in current use can be categorized as TD, including viable vaccines and most of the nonviable vaccines. Only vaccines that contain pure polysaccharide antigens are TI. These include the 23-valent pneumococcal vaccine and the nonviable form of the typhoid vaccine (see **Table 1**). TD vaccines generate more robust responses and long-lived immunologic memory. TI vaccines generate antibody responses that may wane in several years and have very little memory. TI vaccines may be converted into TD vaccines by coupling the target polysaccharide to a protein carrier. These are called "conjugate" vaccines, and the process enhances the otherwise relatively weak immunogenicity of the TI polysaccharide.[5] Conjugate vaccines exist for pneumococcal polysaccharides, *Haemophilus influenzae* type b, and meningococci (see **Table 1**).

DIAGNOSIS OF IMMUNE DEFICIENCY
General Principles

An assessment of humoral immune function is part of the diagnostic evaluation of essentially all patients with suspected immune deficiency.[6–8] For most of these, simple measurement of immunoglobulin isotype levels is not sufficient. Statistically, a small percentage of individuals fall below the lower limit of normal for one or more isotype measurements. Secondary causes may lead to hypogammaglobulinemla (eg, intestinal or renal losses). A functional assessment of antibody production is required to diagnose humoral immune deficiency, unless immunoglobulin is absent. With respect to routine clinical assessment for diagnosing immunodeficiency, the determination of vaccine response measures IgG only.[6-8]

The vaccine response of an individual is assessed with reference to the expected response in the population. "Seroconversion" is the term describing the appearance of a measurable level of immunoglobulin after administration of a vaccine.[1,2] In most cases, the threshold level defining seroconversion is also considered to be the "protective" level of antibody required for vaccine efficacy. Many vaccines have high seroconversion rates (see **Table 1**). Several are less consistently immunogenic, even in a healthy population. Prominent among these are the conjugate and pure polysaccharide vaccines.

TD and TI antigens generate antibody responses via distinct pathways.[4] Some patients with immune deficiency have a relatively selective inability to respond to TI antigens, whereas responses to TD antigens are intact. For example, this is true of patients with specific antibody deficiency with normal immunoglobulins or some patients with common variable immune deficiency. Thus, it is necessary to assess the function of both of these pathways to completely describe the humoral immune competence of an individual.[6-8] Virtually all patients will have had immunization with many TD vaccines at the time of the initial evaluation. Most will not have received any TI (pure polysaccharide) vaccines. To interpret the results of an initial determination of vaccine antibody levels, it is essential to know the immunization history of the patient. Routine immunization schedules may be found on the website of the Centers for Disease Control and Prevention (https://www.cdc.gov/vaccines/schedules/).

TI antigens are poorly immunogenic in young children, and especially so in infants.[9] Readily measurable consistent responses are detected by 1 year of age but continue to improve throughout childhood and into adulthood.[10] It was for this reason that conjugate vaccines for polysaccharide antigens were developed.[11] By joining the polysaccharide to a protein carrier, immunogenicity is greatly enhanced. The introduction of pneumococcal conjugate vaccination in infancy (and adulthood) has led to a significant reduction in the incidence of invasive pneumococcal disease.[12,13] In one meta-analysis encompassing 6,022 immunized children, 26% of children more than 2 years of age with a single episode of invasive pneumococcal infection were diagnosed with an immune deficiency.[14] If more than one invasive pneumococcal infection occurred, the proportion with immune deficiency increased to 67%. The occurrence of invasive pneumococcal infection in an immunized child is an important potential indictor of immune deficiency.

Assessment of T-dependent antibody responses

With respect to TD antigens, measurements of IgG for tetanus (TT) and diphtheria toxoids are used. It is sufficient to measure only one, and TT is most often used.[6-8] There are no data published to indicate that measurement of both is necessary or superior to TT alone. Nor are there data to indicate that measurement of other vaccine responses (eg, measles or polio) are superior, or that measurement of antibodies to multiple TD vaccines enhances diagnostic accuracy. Measurement of TT IgG is appropriate in anyone who has at least completed the primary series of immunizations. This will be the case for most individuals beyond 6 months of age. Functional assessment of humoral immunity in infants less than 6 months old is difficult due to incomplete immunizations, and potential interference by maternal IgG acquired transplacentally during gestation and persistent in the circulation during infancy. If an initial measurement of TT IgG is below the protective threshold (usually 0.15 IU/mL, but it may vary from one laboratory to another), a booster dose should be administered and response assessed 4 weeks later.[6–8] One could consider administering a booster if the level is low (between 0.15 and 1 IU/mL). It is not advisable if the level is higher because (1) the response is probably normal to begin with, and (2) there is increased risk of a large local reaction. Healthy individuals will have a 20- to 30-fold increase in the level of TT IgG.[15] However, clinical laboratories do not routinely report absolute values for levels greater than 7 IU/mL.

Although technically within the TD antigen/vaccine class, conjugate vaccine responses are less commonly used to interrogate humoral immune function.[6–8] The immunogenicity of conjugate vaccines is generally not as consistent as with most other TD vaccines. For *H influenzae* and conjugate pneumococcal vaccines, seroconversion on average is only about 80% in the general population. Normal responses in a healthy population are not well defined, and clinical criteria for diagnosing immunodeficiency using these vaccine responses have not been established. Note also that a small percentage of healthy individuals may not seroconvert to varicella or hepatitis B vaccines.[16,17]

Assessment of T-independent antibody responses

The functional assessment of antibody responses to TI vaccines is much more complex than it is for TD humoral immunity.[6–8] The reason for this is that TI vaccines are not nearly as reliably immunogenic in all ages. Thus, it is difficult to define clearly what constitutes a normal response to a TI vaccine. Responses to pneumococcal polysaccharide vaccines have been studied for decades in both healthy and immunocompromised individuals. Nevertheless, it is not always possible to distinguish impairment of polysaccharide humoral immunity reliably in many cases.

The only pure polysaccharide vaccine in routine use currently is the 23-valent (containing 23 pneumococcal type-specific polysaccharides, **Table 2**) vaccine, PNEUMO-VAX. This is sometimes referred to generically as pneumococcal polysaccharide vaccine (PPSV). This is to be distinguished from the 13-valent pneumococcal conjugate vaccine PREVNAR-13 (generically PCV13). PPSV is in routine clinical use for individuals more than 65 years of age and for younger (19 years and older) individuals at higher risk for invasive pneumococcal disease (eg, with diabetes, chronic heart disease, or chronic obstructive pulmonary disease). Thus, most individuals being evaluated for immune deficiency will never have had this vaccine. However, many will have had previous immunization with PCV13, at least during childhood. (PCV13 came into routine clinical use in 2010. Before that, a 7-valent conjugate pneumococcal vaccine had been in use starting in 2000.) This is important because previous administration of PCV13 can enhance a subsequent response to PPSV. This is called "priming".[18] An individual with poor intrinsic polysaccharide responsiveness may appear to have a more normal response via priming. The duration of the priming effect probably varies from one individual to another. At least 1 year is likely for most individuals; it may be longer for some. Note that previous immunization with PPSV may lead to a modest reduction in the subsequent response to PCV or additional doses of PPSV.[19] This inhibitory effect may also last approximately 1 year.

It is appropriate to use PPSV to evaluate the capacity to produce antibody to pure polysaccharide (TI antigen). The PCV, as a conjugate vaccine, represents a TD antigen, and should not be used for this purpose.[6–8] A dose of PPSV is given and the response is measured 4 weeks later. Ideally, pre- and post-immunization sera are analyzed together, but this is not done routinely in clinical practice. Measurements

Table 2
Serotypes contained in pneumococcal vaccines

Serotype Designations[a]

US System	Danish System	Prevnar	Prevnar 13	Pneumovax 23
1	1		X	X
2	2			X
3	3		X	X
4	4	X	X	X
5	5		X	X
6	6A		X	
7	7F		X	X
8	8			X
9	9N			X
12	12F			X
14	14	X	X	X
17	17F			X
19	19F	X	X	X
20	20			X
22	22F			X
23	23F	X	X	X
26	6B	X	X	X
33	33F			X
34	10A			X
43	11A			X
54	15B			X
56	18C	X	X	X
57	19A		X	X
68	9V	X	X	X

[a] There are two systems of nomenclature for pneumococcal serotypes: the system of the United States and the Danish system.

should at least be conducted in the same laboratory. Levels of IgG for each of the 23 serotypes in PPSV are measured, often simultaneously with determination of immunoglobulin isotypes and TT IgG. If the patient has received a recent (within 1–2 years) dose of PCV, attention should be focused on serotypes found only in PPSV, to avoid confounding the interpretation due to the effect of priming. If PCV had been given more remotely, one may include all 23 types in the analysis. If levels for most serotypes are low (approximately <1–2 μg/mL), the vaccine is given and the response is assessed. If levels are higher for many serotypes, the vaccine should be given with caution, because there may be greater risk for a severe local reaction.

As already noted, the interpretation of PPSV response is not straightforward. The most widely cited figure for the threshold for protection with respect to a single serotype after pure polysaccharide is 1.3 μg/mL.[20] The validity of this threshold value has been questioned.[21] Note also that the established criterion for protection after pneumococcal conjugate vaccine is 0.35 μg/mL.[20,21] It is not necessarily the case that one threshold is correct and the other is not. The vaccines stimulate antibody responses differently; the isotype profiles of the responses are different and likely differ in affinity/avidity as well.

Criteria for fold increase in level according to age as well as persistence of antibody in the circulation have been proposed (**Table 3**). However, these statements represent at best a rough guide. Sensitivity and (especially) specificity, somewhat loosely defined in this context, are poor.[22] In some studies using fifth percentile cutoffs for pneumococcal serotype, specific measurements perform better than the criteria in **Table 3**. However, many laboratories do not report percentile ranges or cutoffs for these measurements.[22] These considerations of varying concentration and fold-increase thresholds of protection after administration of different types of vaccine challenge attempts to apply proposed criteria for immune deficiency diagnosis in a systematic way.

Alternative or complementary measurements of other polysaccharide responses have been proposed in attempts to increase diagnostic accuracy. For example, responses to *Salmonella typhi* pure polysaccharide vaccine have been studied.[22–25] Measurement of typhoid polysaccharide vaccine response performs at least as well as PPSV clinically and has the advantages of being simpler (a single measurement instead of measuring responses to many pneumococcal types), and suitable for patients who are on IgG therapy, because therapeutic IgG does not contain *S typhi* antibody. In this regard, *S typhi* vaccine performs as a neoantigen (see later). However, most clinical reference laboratories do not yet offer measurement of *S typhi* IgG, and this has not yet been incorporated into guidelines for immune deficiency evaluation.

Clinical evaluation of humoral immune function to date has focused exclusively on antibody quantity: the serum concentration of antibody produced after immunization. This completely ignores the critical dimensions of antibody quality. The latter refers to several biologic properties such as (1) the affinity or avidity of the antibody, the strength of the binding to its antigen, (2) the isotype profile, and (3) other antibody characteristics that have an impact on the ability to activate complement and opsonophagocytic activity via IgG Fc receptors and/or complement. Methodologies exist to measure these aspects of antibody function, but none are established for routine clinical use and criteria defining the spectrum of normal antibody functions are not well established.[26,27] This is important because it has become clear that some (perhaps many) individuals may express clinical humoral immune deficiency due to poor antibody quality although they produce normal-appearing quantities of antibodies.[28–30]

Table 3
Phenotypes for specific antibody deficiency based on responsiveness to PPSV

Phenotype	Age <6 y	Age >6 y
Mild	Concentration <1.3 μg/mL for multiple serotypes, or 2-fold increase for <50% of serotypes	Concentration <1.3 μg/mL for multiple serotypes, or 2-fold increase for <70% of serotypes
Moderate	Concentration >1.3 μg/mL for <50% of serotypes	Concentration >1.3 μg/mL for <70% of serotypes
Severe	Concentration >1.3 μg/mL for ≤2 serotypes	
Memory	Loss of response within 6 mo	

From Orange JS, Ballow M, Stiehm ER, et al. Use and interpretation of diagnostic vaccination in primary immunodeficiency: a working group report of the Basic and Clinical Immunology Interest Section of the American Academy of Allergy, Asthma & Immunology. J Allergy Clin Immunol 2012;130(3 Suppl):S14; with permission.

Patients Receiving IgG Therapy

It is sometimes desired to assess humoral immune function in patients receiving IgG replacement therapy. This may be to confirm a diagnosis in a patient who may not have had a thorough assessment before initiating therapy, or to know if it is likely to be safe to discontinue therapy in an individual whose immune deficiency may not be permanent as in secondary immune deficiency or transient hypogammaglobulinemia of infancy. This is not possible with most TD vaccine responses because therapeutic IgG contains high levels of most of these antibodies. In this setting, it may be useful to measure a response to a so-called neoantigen; an immunogen not previously encountered by the patient and one for which antibodies are not generally found in therapeutic IgG.

Research studies have used bacteriophage phi-X174 as such a neoantigen.[31] Both primary (IgM) and secondary (IgG) responses may be assessed. Keyhole limpet hemocyanin has also been studied in this way.[32] Neither of these modalities is readily applicable for general clinical use. A few reports have shown the utility of rabies virus vaccine as a neoantigen in immune-deficient patients.[8,33] This could be used clinically because both the vaccine and measurement of rabies IgG are readily available. Furthermore, rabies virus IgG is not measurable in therapeutic IgG.

Similarly, PPSV is not suitable for measurement of a TI antibody response in patients receiving IgG, because these antibodies are well represented in therapeutic IgG. For this purpose, S typhi polysaccharide vaccine could be used.[23]

THERAPY OF IMMUNE DEFICIENCY

Almost all patients with immune deficiency will have received several vaccines before diagnosis. Exceptions include those diagnosed prenatally or at birth due to family history, or those diagnosed with T cell defects via newborn screening for severe combined immune deficiency. The risk/benefit calculation for vaccine use in patients with immune deficiency is different from that for normal individuals and depends largely on the specific immune deficiency disorder under consideration.[34] Killed or subcomponent vaccines are generally safe for all forms of immune deficiency, because they cannot cause disease. However, for defects that include some component of impaired specific immunity, the benefit is usually minimal, because antibody response is minimal or absent. However, patients with phagocytic cell defects or complement defects and many innate defects should receive all of these vaccines, because they will produce antibody in most circumstances.

Patients who are receiving IgG will not need immunization with most inactivated vaccines, because antibodies against these organisms are usually well represented in therapeutic IgG. Exceptions include hepatitis A, human papilloma virus, influenza virus, and meningococcus. These vaccines should be given according to the routine schedule unless it is deemed that there is no possibility of response. Responses to some of these vaccines have been studied in patients with humoral immune deficiency receiving IgG. Among 23 patients with common variable immunodeficiency (CVID) on IgG who received tetanus and diphtheria toxoids, H influenzae conjugate, hepatitis A and B, and pneumococcal polysaccharide, 18% to 23% of patients had measurable responses.[35] Another study documented good responses to meningococcal polysaccharide vaccine in up to 65% of 23 patients with CVID on IgG.[36] Note that the meningococcal polysaccharide vaccine is no longer in use; it has been replaced with conjugate-type vaccines. Theoretically at least, these would also be expected to be immunogenic in this setting.

Human papillomavirus vaccine may be of specific utility in disorders with increased susceptibility to these viruses.[37] These include severe combined immunodeficiency (SCID), Wiskott-Aldrich syndrome, ataxia-telangiectasia, NF-kappa B essential modulator (NEMO) deficiency, leukocyte adhesion deficiency (CD18 mutation), X-linked hyper-IgM syndrome, WILD syndrome (disseminated warts, immunodeficiency, lymphedema, anogenital dysplasia), epidermodysplasia verruciformis (mutations of TMC6 or TMC8), GATA2 deficiency, WHIM syndrome (warts, hypogammaglobulinemia, infections, myelokathexis, CXCR5 mutation), autosomal recessive hyper-IgE syndrome (DOCK8 mutation), Netherton syndrome (SPINK5 mutation), and MST1 and RhoH mutations.

An injectable form of influenza vaccine is generally recommended annually for all patients with primary immune deficiency.[34,38] Response to influenza vaccine has been studied in patients with humoral immune defects.[39] Response was detected in most, although at a protective level only for approximately 20%. Cellular immune responses are also diminished in these patients.[40] In addition to immunization, medication prophylaxis may also be used to prevent influenza morbidity.

Much more caution is required with the use of any form of viable vaccine, because there may be significant risk of disease caused by the vaccine organism (see later). In general, these vaccines should be avoided in any patients with severe defects of T cell function, severe antibody deficiency, or diseases that are associated with increased susceptibility to viral infections.[34] Conversely, measles-mumps-rubella (MMR) vaccine should be given to patients with milder T cell defects (see criteria for live vaccines in DiGeorge syndrome), most phagocytic cell disorders (possibly excepting leukocyte adhesion deficiency), complement defects, autoinflammatory disorders, diseases of immune dysregulation, and innate defects not predisposing to viral infections. There are no reported cases of vaccine measles transmission to immune-deficient household contacts of vaccines, so this should not be a concern. On the contrary, measles immunization of household contacts of immune-compromised individuals is strongly recommended to protect them from exposure to wild-type virus (see https://www.cdc.gov/vaccines/vpd/mmr/hcp/recommendations.html).

In patients receiving IgG, the most commonly used viable vaccines are not needed, because antibodies are well represented in therapeutic IgG. Prominent among these are MMR and varicella/zoster vaccines.[34] These vaccines are specifically contraindicated in patients receiving IgG, because they are neutralized by antibodies in therapeutic IgG.[41]

ADVERSE EFFECTS OF VACCINES IN PATIENTS WITH IMMUNE DEFICIENCY

Significant adverse consequences of vaccines in patients with immune deficiency are limited to those containing viable organisms. These may range from mild to fatal. Thus, there must be careful assessment of potential benefit versus risk regarding use of these vaccines in this population.

Measles-Mumps-Rubella and Varicella Vaccines

These vaccines, especially varicella, have long been known to be potential causes of serious disease and death in patients with severe T cell defects.[42-45] They are usually well tolerated in patients with milder T cell defects, such as DiGeorge syndrome.[46-49] However, some patients with DiGeorge syndrome have severely impaired T cell function and are at risk for complications from these vaccines.[50,51] Published criteria for safe administration of live vaccines in DiGeorge syndrome include (1) adequate response to nonviable vaccines, (2) normal or near-normal in vitro T cell response to mitogens and recall antigens, (3) CD8 T cell count greater than 300 cells/mm^3, and (4) a CD4 cell count greater than 500 cells/mm^3.[46,52]

Vaccine strain rubella is increasingly recognized as causing indolent persistent infection in patients with impaired cellular immunity.[53–55] Cutaneous and visceral granulomatous lesions have been found in patients with a variety of immune defects, including ataxia-telangiectasia, ARTEMIS deficiency, cartilage-hair hypoplasia, Coronin-1a deficiency, DNA ligase 4 deficiency, MHC Class II deficiency, Nijmegen breakage syndrome, WHIM syndrome, and X-linked SCID. Replicating rubella virus has been recovered from some of these lesions. Shedding of infectious virus from skin lesions could pose a risk to unimmunized contacts.[56] Most of these diagnoses would not necessarily be suspected at the time of routine MMR administration. The only consistently effective therapy has been stem cell transplantation, although some have been reported to clear with steroids or anti-tumor necrosis factor agents.[57]

Oral Polio Vaccine

Oral polio vaccine was among the earliest recognized to cause severe disease in patients with impaired cellular and/or humoral immune function.[58] This led to the exclusive use of inactivated polio vaccine for the primary series of immunizations in many countries. However, use of oral polio vaccine is still widespread throughout the world, and the administration of this vaccine to immunocompromised hosts may be hindering efforts to eradicate the disease.[59–63] The vaccine strain polio virus can persist and be excreted for years to cause disease in unimmunized contacts. Such reported cases are rare (approximately 1.3 cases per year total from 26 countries surveyed in one study[59]), but this may underestimate the actual number of cases of transmission.[64]

Rotavirus Vaccine

Rotavirus vaccine is a combination of elements from human and bovine strains. Soon after its introduction in 2006, it was reported to cause diarrheal disease in infants with severe combined immune deficiency.[65,66] Reports continue to accumulate, but no deaths have yet been reported.[67,68] Infections resolve with stem cell therapy. This is currently the only viable vaccine that is part of the routine infant immunization series in North America. Newborn screening for SCID will mitigate the potential for these occurrences.[69,70]

Bacille Calmette-Guerin

Bacille Calmette-Guerin (BCG) is the only mycobacterial vaccine in current use; it is a bovine strain (*Mycobacterium bovis*) administered to protect against disease caused by *Mycobacterium tuberculosis*. The vaccine is used throughout the world with the exception of North America, most of Europe, Scandinavia, Ecuador, and Australia.[71] Note that not all countries use the same strain of *M bovis* for vaccination; strains differ in their immunogenicity and their potential to cause disease in immunocompromised hosts. BCG is responsible for approximately 75% of the adverse effects of live agent immunization in immune-deficient patients in one center.[72] Not surprisingly, patients with SCID are highly susceptible to infections with this vaccine. Interestingly, forms of SCID where natural killer cell function is absent (X-linked SCID, Jak3 deficiency, reticular dysgenesis, and adenosine deaminase deficiency) are particularly susceptible.[73] Also susceptible are those with any of a group of disorders referred to as Mendelian susceptibility to mycobacterial disease, such as defects of the interleukin-12/interferon-gamma axis.[74–77] A number of fatalities due to disseminated infection have been reported. Severe adenopathy in draining nodes of vaccination sites is a possible indicator of immune deficiency.[77] A family history of complications of BCG immunization should also be sought before administration of the vaccine.[78]

DISCLOSURE

F.A. Bonilla has been a speaker for Takeda Pharmaceutical Co, Ltd.

REFERENCES

1. Bester JC. Measles and measles vaccination: a review. JAMA Pediatr 2016; 170(12):1209–15.
2. Siegrist C-A. Vaccine immunology. In: Plotkin SA, Orenstein WA, Offit PA, editors. Vaccines. 6th edition. Philadelphia: WB Saunders; 2012. p. 14–32.
3. The history of vaccines. 2020. Available at: https://www.historyofvaccines.org/. Accessed January 4, 2020.
4. Bonilla FA, Oettgen HC. Adaptive immunity. J Allergy Clin Immunol 2010;125(2 Suppl 2):S33–40.
5. Moens L, Picard C, Shahrooei M, et al. Different immunological pathways underlie the immune response to pneumococcal polysaccharides. J Clin Immunol 2017; 37(3):277–8.
6. Ballow M. Use of vaccines In the evaluation of presumed immunodeficiency. Ann Allergy Asthma Immunol 2013;111(3):163–6.
7. Bonilla FA, Khan DA, Ballas ZK, et al. Practice parameter for the diagnosis and management of primary immunodeficiency. J Allergy Clin Immunol 2015;136(5): 1186–205.e1-78.
8. Orange JS, Ballow M, Stiehm ER, et al. Use and interpretation of diagnostic vaccination in primary immunodeficiency: a working group report of the Basic and Clinical Immunology Interest Section of the American Academy of Allergy, Asthma & Immunology. J Allergy Clin Immunol 2012;130(3 Suppl):S1–24.
9. Koskela M, Leinonen M, Haiva VM, et al. First and second dose antibody responses to pneumococcal polysaccharide vaccine in infants. Pediatr Infect Dis 1986;5(1):45–50.
10. Bossuyt X, Borgers H, Moens L, et al. Age- and serotype-dependent antibody response to pneumococcal polysaccharides. J Allergy Clin Immunol 2011; 127(4):1079–80 [author reply: 1080–1].
11. Payton T, Girgenti D, Frenck RW, et al. Immunogenicity, safety, and tolerability of three lots of 13-valent pneumococcal conjugate vaccine given with routine pediatric vaccinations in the United States. Pediatr Infect Dis J 2013;32(8):871–80.
12. Dondo V, Mujuru H, Nathoo K, et al. Pneumococcal conjugate vaccine impact on meningitis and pneumonia among children aged <5 years - Zimbabwe, 2010-2016. Clin Infect Dis 2019;69(Supplement_2):S72–80.
13. Johnstone SL, Moore DP, Klugman KP, et al. Epidemiology of invasive bacterial infections in pneumococcal conjugate vaccine-vaccinated and -unvaccinated children under 5 years of age in Soweto, South Africa: a cohort study from a high-HIV burden setting. Paediatr Int Child Health 2020;40(1):50–7.
14. Butters C, Phuong LK, Cole T, et al. Prevalence of immunodeficiency in children with invasive pneumococcal disease in the pneumococcal vaccine era: a systematic review. JAMA Pediatr 2019. https://doi.org/10.1001/jamapediatrics.2019. 3203.
15. McCusker C, Somerville W, Grey V, et al. Specific antibody responses to diphtheria/tetanus revaccination in children evaluated for immunodeficiency. Ann Allergy Asthma Immunol 1997;79(2):145–50.

16. Michalik DE, Steinberg SP, Larussa PS, et al. Primary vaccine failure after 1 dose of varicella vaccine in healthy children. J Infect Dis 2008;197(7):944–9.

17. Shokri F, Amani A. High rate of seroconversion following administration of a single supplementary dose of recombinant hepatitis B vaccine in Iranian healthy nonresponder neonates. Med Microbiol Immunol 1997;185(4):231–5.

18. Schaballie H, Wuyts G, Dillaerts D, et al. Effect of previous vaccination with pneumococcal conjugate vaccine on pneumococcal polysaccharide vaccine antibody responses. Clin Exp Immunol 2016;185(2):180–9.

19. O'Brien KL, Hochman M, Goldblatt D. Combined schedules of pneumococcal conjugate and polysaccharide vaccines: is hyporesponsiveness an issue? Lancet Infect Dis 2007;7(9):597–606.

20. Sorensen RU, Edgar D. Specific antibody deficiencies in clinical practice. J Allergy Clin Immunol Pract 2019;7(3):801–8.

21. McNulty CMG, Li JT. Interpretation of post-pneumococcal vaccine antibody levels: concerns and pitfalls. J Allergy Clin Immunol Pract 2019;7(3):1061–2.

22. Schaballie H, Bosch B, Schrijvers R, et al. Fifth percentile cutoff values for anti-pneumococcal polysaccharide and anti-salmonella typhi Vi IgG describe a normal polysaccharide response. Front Immunol 2017;8:546.

23. Bausch-Jurken MT, Verbsky JW, Gonzaga KA, et al. The use of salmonella typhim vaccine to diagnose antibody deficiency. J Clin Immunol 2017;37(5):427–33.

24. Evans C, Bateman E, Steven R, et al. Measurement of Typhi Vi antibodies can be used to assess adaptive immunity in patients with immunodeficiency. Clin Exp Immunol 2018;192(3):292–301.

25. Guevara-Hoyer K, Gil C, Parker AR, et al. Measurement of Typhim Vi IgG as a diagnostic tool to determine anti-polysaccharide antibody production deficiency in children. Front Immunol 2019;10:654.

26. Fried AJ, Altrich ML, Liu H, et al. Correlation of pneumococcal antibody concentration and avidity with patient clinical and immunologic characteristics. J Clin Immunol 2013;33(4):847–56.

27. LaFon DC, Nahm MH. Measuring immune responses to pneumococcal vaccines. J Immunol Methods 2018;461:37–43.

28. Romero-Steiner S, Frasch CE, Carlone G, et al. Use of opsonophagocytosis for serological evaluation of pneumococcal vaccines. Clin Vaccin Immunol 2006; 13(2):165–9.

29. Rose CE, Romero-Steiner S, Burton RL, et al. Multilaboratory comparison of Streptococcus pneumoniae opsonophagocytic killing assays and their level of agreement for the determination of functional antibody activity in human reference sera. Clin Vaccin Immunol 2011;18(1):135–42.

30. Whaley MJ, Rose C, Martinez J, et al. Interlaboratory comparison of three multiplexed bead-based immunoassays for measuring serum antibodies to pneumococcal polysaccharides. Clin Vaccin Immunol 2010;17(5):862–9.

31. Ochs HD, Buckley RH, Kobayashi RH, et al. Antibody responses to bacteriophage phi X174 in patients with adenosine deaminase deficiency. Blood 1992; 80(5):1163–71.

32. Kondratenko I, Amlot PL, Webster AD, et al. Lack of specific antibody response in common variable immunodeficiency (CVID) associated with failure in production of antigen-specific memory T cells. MRC Immunodeficiency Group. Clin Exp Immunol 1997;108(1):9–13.

33. van Zelm MC, Reisli I, van der Burg M, et al. An antibody-deficiency syndrome due to mutations in the CD19 gene. N Engl J Med 2006;354(18):1901–12.

34. Sobh A, Bonilla FA. Vaccination in primary immunodeficiency disorders. J Allergy Clin Immunol Pract 2016;4(6):1066–75.
35. Goldacker S, Draeger R, Warnatz K, et al. Active vaccination in patients with common variable immunodeficiency (CVID). Clin Immunol 2007;124(3):294–303.
36. Rezaei N, Siadat SD, Aghamohammadi A, et al. Serum bactericidal antibody response 1 year after meningococcal polysaccharide vaccination of patients with common variable immunodeficiency. Clin Vaccin Immunol 2010;17(4):524–8.
37. Leiding JW, Holland SM. Warts and all: human papillomavirus in primary immunodeficiencies. J Allergy Clin Immunol 2012;130(5):1030–48.
38. Junker AK, Bonilla FA, Sullivan KE. How to flee the flu. Clin Immunol 2004;112(3):219–20.
39. van Assen S, Holvast A, Telgt DS, et al. Patients with humoral primary immunodeficiency do not develop protective anti-influenza antibody titers after vaccination with trivalent subunit influenza vaccine. Clin Immunol 2010;136(2):228–35.
40. van Assen S, de Haan A, Holvast A, et al. Cell-mediated immune responses to inactivated trivalent influenza-vaccination are decreased in patients with common variable immunodeficiency. Clin Immunol 2011;141(2):161–8.
41. Medical Advisory Committee of the Immune Deficiency Foundation, Shearer WT, Fleisher TA, et al. Recommendations for live viral and bacterial vaccines in immunodeficient patients and their close contacts. J Allergy Clin Immunol 2014;133(4):961–6.
42. Bayer DK, Martinez CA, Sorte HS, et al. Vaccine-associated varicella and rubella infections in severe combined immunodeficiency with isolated CD4 lymphocytopenia and mutations in IL7R detected by tandem whole exome sequencing and chromosomal microarray. Clin Exp Immunol 2014;178(3):459–69.
43. Bitnun A, Shannon P, Durward A, et al. Measles inclusion-body encephalitis caused by the vaccine strain of measles virus. Clin Infect Dis 1999;29(4):855–61.
44. Leung J, Siegel S, Jones JF, et al. Fatal varicella due to the vaccine-strain varicella-zoster virus. Hum Vaccin Immunother 2014;10(1):146–9.
45. Schuil J, van de Putte EM, Zwaan CM, et al. Retinopathy following measles, mumps, and rubella vaccination in an immuno-incompetent girl. Int Ophthalmol 1998;22(6):345–7.
46. Al-Sukaiti N, Reid B, Lavi S, et al. Safety and efficacy of measles, mumps, and rubella vaccine in patients with DiGeorge syndrome. J Allergy Clin Immunol 2010;126(4):868–9.
47. Azzari C, Gambineri E, Resti M, et al. Safety and immunogenicity of measles-mumps-rubella vaccine in children with congenital immunodeficiency (DiGeorge syndrome). Vaccine 2005;23(14):1668–71.
48. Hofstetter AM, Jakob K, Klein NP, et al. Live vaccine use and safety in DiGeorge syndrome. Pediatrics 2014;133(4):e946–54.
49. Perez EE, Bokszczanin A, McDonald-McGinn D, et al. Safety of live viral vaccines in patients with chromosome 22q11.2 deletion syndrome (DiGeorge syndrome/velocardiofacial syndrome). Pediatrics 2003;112(4):e325.
50. Valenzise M, Cascio A, Wasniewska M, et al. Post vaccine acute disseminated encephalomyelitis as the first manifestation of chromosome 22q11.2 deletion syndrome in a 15-month old baby: a case report. Vaccine 2014;32(43):5552–4.
51. Waters V, Peterson KS, LaRussa P. Live viral vaccines in a DiGeorge syndrome patient. Arch Dis Child 2007;92(6):519–20.
52. Sullivan KE. DiGeorge syndrome and chromosome 22q11.2 deletion syndrome. In: Ochs HD, Stiehm ER, Winkelstein JA, editors. Immunologic disorders in infants and children. 5 edition. Philadelphia: Elsevier; 2004. p. 523–38.

53. Bodemer C, Sauvage V, Mahlaoui N, et al. Live rubella virus vaccine long-term persistence as an antigenic trigger of cutaneous granulomas in patients with primary immunodeficiency. Clin Microbiol Infect 2014;20(10):O656–63.

54. Perelygina L, Buchbinder D, Dorsey MJ, et al. Outcomes for nitazoxanide treatment in a case series of patients with primary immunodeficiencies and rubella virus-associated granuloma. J Clin Immunol 2019;39(1):112–7.

55. Murguia-Favela L, Hiebert J, Haber RM. "Noninfectious" cutaneous granulomas in primary immunodeficiency patients and association with rubella virus vaccine strain. J Cutan Med Surg 2019;23(3):341–2.

56. Perelygina L, Chen MH, Suppiah S, et al. Infectious vaccine-derived rubella viruses emerge, persist, and evolve in cutaneous granulomas of children with primary immunodeficiencies. PLoS Pathog 2019;15(10):e1008080.

57. Buchbinder D, Hauck F, Albert MH, et al. Rubella virus-associated cutaneous granulomatous disease: a unique complication in immune-deficient patients, not limited to DNA repair disorders. J Clin Immunol 2019;39(1):81–9.

58. Hara M, Saito Y, Komatsu T, et al. Antigenic analysis of polioviruses isolated from a child with agammaglobulinemia and paralytic poliomyelitis after Sabin vaccine administration. Microbiol Immunol 1981;25(9):905–13.

59. Guo J, Bolivar-Wagers S, Srinivas N, et al. Immunodeficiency-related vaccine-derived poliovirus (iVDPV) cases: a systematic review and implications for polio eradication. Vaccine 2015;33(10):1235–42.

60. Jorba J, Diop OM, Iber J, et al. Update on vaccine-derived polioviruses - worldwide, January 2015-May 2016. MMWR Morb Mortal Wkly Rep 2016;65(30):763–9.

61. Li L, Ivanova O, Driss N, et al. Poliovirus excretion among persons with primary immune deficiency disorders: summary of a seven-country study series. J Infect Dis 2014;210(Suppl 1):S368–72.

62. Kalkowska DA, Pallansch MA, Thompson KM. Updated modelling of the prevalence of immunodeficiency-associated long-term vaccine-derived poliovirus (iVDPV) excreters. Epidemiol Infect 2019;147:e295.

63. Weil M, Rahav G, Somech R, et al. First report of a persistent oropharyngeal infection of type 2 vaccine-derived poliovirus (iVDPV2) in a primary immune deficient (PID) patient after eradication of wild type 2 poliovirus. Int J Infect Dis 2019; 83:40–3.

64. Shaghaghi M, Shahmahmoodi S, Nili A, et al. Vaccine-derived poliovirus infection among patients with primary immunodeficiency and effect of patient screening on disease outcomes, Iran. Emerg Infect Dis 2019;25(11):2005–12.

65. Kaplon J, Cros G, Ambert-Balay K, et al. Rotavirus vaccine virus shedding, viremia and clearance in infants with severe combined immune deficiency. Pediatr Infect Dis J 2015;34(3):326–8.

66. Patel NC, Hertel PM, Estes MK, et al. Vaccine-acquired rotavirus in infants with severe combined immunodeficiency. N Engl J Med 2010;362(4):314–9.

67. Chiu M, Bao C, Sadarangani M. Dilemmas with rotavirus vaccine: the neonate and immunocompromised. Pediatr Infect Dis J 2019;38(6S Suppl 1):S43–6.

68. Yoshikawa T, Ihira M, Higashimoto Y, et al. Persistent systemic rotavirus vaccine infection in a child with X-linked severe combined immunodeficiency. J Med Virol 2019;91(6):1008–13.

69. De Francesco MA, Ianiro G, Monini M, et al. Persistent infection with rotavirus vaccine strain in severe combined immunodeficiency (SCID) child: is rotavirus vaccination in SCID children a Janus face? Vaccines (Basel) 2019;7(4) [pii:E185].

70. Gower CM, Dunning J, Nawaz S, et al. Vaccine-derived rotavirus strains in infants in England. Arch Dis Child 2019. https://doi.org/10.1136/archdischild-2019-317428.
71. BCG world atlas. 2017; 2. Available at: http://www.bcgatlas.org/. Accessed January 12, 2020.
72. Sarmiento JD, Villada F, Orrego JC, et al. Adverse events following immunization in patients with primary immunodeficiencies. Vaccine 2016;34(13):1611–6.
73. Bernatowska E, Skomska-Pawliszak M, Wolska-Kusnierz B, et al. BCG Moreau vaccine safety profile and NK cells-double protection against disseminated BCG infection in retrospective study of BCG vaccination in 52 Polish children with severe combined immunodeficiency. J Clin Immunol 2019;40(1):138–46.
74. Bernatowska EA, Wolska-Kusnierz B, Pac M, et al. Disseminated bacillus Calmette-Guerin infection and immunodeficiency. Emerg Infect Dis 2007;13(5): 799–801.
75. Boudjemaa S, Dainese L, Heritier S, et al. Disseminated bacillus Calmette-Guerin osteomyelitis in twin sisters related to STAT1 gene deficiency. Pediatr Dev Pathol 2017;20(3):255–61.
76. Marciano BE, Huang CY, Joshi G, et al. BCG vaccination in patients with severe combined immunodeficiency: complications, risks, and vaccination policies. J Allergy Clin Immunol 2014;133(4):1134–41.
77. Santos A, Dias A, Cordeiro A, et al. Severe axillary lymphadenitis after BCG vaccination: alert for primary immunodeficiencies. J Microbiol Immunol Infect 2010;43(6):530–7.
78. Roxo-Junior P, Silva J, Andrea M, et al. A family history of serious complications due to BCG vaccination is a tool for the early diagnosis of severe primary immunodeficiency. Ital J Pediatr 2013;39:54.

Chronic Lung Disease in Primary Antibody Deficiency
Diagnosis and Management

Paul J. Maglione, MD, PhD

KEYWORDS

- Primary antibody deficiency • Common variable immunodeficiency • Lung disease
- Asthma • Bronchiectasis • Interstitial lung disease • GLILD

KEY POINTS

- Chronic lung disease is a frequent complication of primary antibody deficiency that can manifest in numerous distinct forms.
- Asthma and chronic obstructive pulmonary disease are common forms of lung disease with unique considerations relating to pathogenesis and treatment when they occur in PAD.
- Bronchiectasis development and progression are linked with delayed diagnosis and inadequate treatment of PAD, but can still worsen despite prophylactic measures to limit infection.
- Interstitial lung disease is associated with high morbidity and mortality in PAD and results from pulmonary lymphoproliferative pathology that is responsive to immunomodulatory therapy.

INTRODUCTION

Primary antibody deficiency (PAD) is the most commonly diagnosed inborn error of immunity, consisting of numerous conditions in which impairment of immunoglobulin production is the dominant phenotype.[1] PAD consists of a spectrum of clinical phenotypes from the relatively mild, such as selective immunoglobulin A (IgA) deficiency (IgAD), to those with severe antibody loss, as in X-linked agammaglobulinemia (XLA).[2] The most prevalent symptomatic form of PAD is common variable immunodeficiency (CVID), which is defined by profoundly low IgG and IgA and/or IgM as well as failure to mount antibodies against vaccination.[3] Because CVID is the most frequently encountered, most studies of PAD and lung disease have focused on this diagnosis.[4] Recognition of PAD is often delayed by many years, which may increase the risk of chronic lung disease.[5]

Pulmonary Center, Boston University School of Medicine, 72 East Concord Street, R304, Boston, MA 02118, USA
E-mail address: pmaglion@bu.edu

Immunol Allergy Clin N Am 40 (2020) 437–459
https://doi.org/10.1016/j.iac.2020.03.003
0889-8561/20/© 2020 Elsevier Inc. All rights reserved.
immunology.theclinics.com

Evaluation of PAD is most frequently preceded by a history of recurrent acute respiratory infections, often of bacterial etiology.[6,7] Frequent and/or severe respiratory infections can cause structural lung damage that may promote chronic pulmonary disease.[8] Moreover, delay in PAD diagnosis is associated with fixed pulmonary obstruction, chronic atelectasis, pulmonary fibrosis, and bronchiectasis.[6,9,10] Earlier recognition of PAD potentially can lead to interventions that reduce the frequency of respiratory infections, hospital admissions, and improve survival.[11–13] It is widely accepted that the infection susceptibility in PAD stems from loss of the important contribution of antibodies in immunity against bacteria.[14] Supporting this concept, encapsulated bacteria, for which immunity is thought to be particularly reliant on antibodies, are the most frequently cultured pathogens from sputum of patients with PAD.[15,16] Efficacy of antibiotic prophylaxis for reduction of annual respiratory exacerbations in patients with PAD was recently demonstrated in a large placebo-controlled trial, resulting in encouragingly low levels of antibiotic resistance.[17] In addition to bacteria, viruses are also frequent instigators of respiratory disease in PAD and should not be overlooked.[18–20]

Despite improved recognition of PAD and management of acute respiratory infections in these patients, chronic lung disease still occurs frequently and pulmonary function declines over time.[21] In a single-center study of 473 patients with CVID, functional or structural lung impairment was reported in 28.5% of subjects, with significantly reduced survival compared with patients with CVID without chronic lung disease.[22] Lower respiratory tract infections with encapsulated bacteria may be of particular importance to the development of chronic lung disease as *H influenzae* and *S pneumoniae* have been shown to lead to pleurisy, empyema, and bronchospasm in CVID.[23] It seems that early intervention with prophylactic antibiotics and/or immunoglobulin replacement therapy (IRT) can reduce respiratory infections and decrease morbidity and mortality from pulmonary disease in PAD.[11,12,24–27] However, chronic lung disease progresses in many patients with PAD despite widespread usage of antibiotic prophylaxis and IRT.[28–30] This may be explained, at least in part, by immune dysregulation occurring independent of infection.[31] Alternatively, there may be important host defense mechanisms that remain deficient despite IRT, such as mucosal IgM and IgA responses. Infection-driven and noninfection-driven pathways of chronic lung disease alike must be better understood in order to improve care of PAD.

One particularly interesting observation that demonstrates the complexity of lung disease susceptibility in patients with PAD is that respiratory infections and chronic lung disease occurs more frequently in those with CVID compared with XLA, despite XLA resulting in more profound antibody deficiency.[32,33] Comparison of CVID and XLA suggests that differences in genetic etiology, concurrent T-cell defects, propensity for immune dysregulation, and/or differences in diagnostic delay may explain why these 2 forms of severe PAD have differing prevalence of lung disease.[33] For example, PAD with concurrent disruption of T-cell function, such as hyper IgM syndrome due to defects of CD40:CD40 L interaction, can lead to a broader range of respiratory pathogens, including *Histoplasma* and *Pneumocystis*.[34] Although increased susceptibility to respiratory infections and chronic lung disease is shared among the diverse forms of PAD, immunologic differences shape individual variations in pulmonary manifestations.

Key points regarding respiratory infections in PAD are highlighted in **Box 1**. As with many chronic diseases, thoughtful clinical surveillance and intervention is vital for management of lung disease in PAD. Unfortunately, there is significant variance among physicians regarding follow-up and monitoring of respiratory disease in

---

Box 1
Key points regarding respiratory infection in patients with PAD

- Encapsulated bacteria are the most common pathogens isolated from the respiratory tract of patients with PAD, but viruses are also frequent and may be underappreciated in importance.

- Prophylactic antibiotics can be used to reduce the frequency of respiratory infections in patients with PAD without a significant increase in antibiotic resistance.

- Chronic lung disease develops in some patients with PAD despite improved recognition of immune deficiency and usage of IRT.

- Chronic lung disease may develop because of immune dysregulation independent of infection or deficiencies in host defense that are not alleviated by IRT and/or antibiotic prophylaxis.

PAD.[35] Appropriate usage of chest imaging and pulmonary function testing (PFT) forms the basis of the diagnostic work-up of a patient with PAD with suspected chronic lung disease, with tissue biopsy used when indicated. Therapeutic response, or lack thereof, often provides an additional modality of clinical evaluation. Emerging diagnostic tools and precision medical therapies are dramatically altering the landscape of lung disease management in PAD. Specific diagnostic and therapeutic concerns applicable to common forms of chronic lung disease affecting patients with PAD will now be explored further.

ASTHMA AND CHRONIC OBSTRUCTIVE PULMONARY DISEASE

Asthma and chronic obstructive pulmonary disease (COPD) are common forms of chronic lung disease in the general population that also frequently affect those with PAD. These are obstructive forms of lung disease resulting from airway constriction owing, at least in part, to chronic inflammation. Depending on the cohort studied, obstructive lung disease, or at least bronchial hyperresponsiveness, has been reported in 15% to 50% of those with CVID and at least 5% of patients with XLA.[36–38] Leveraging the United States Immunodeficiency Network we found further evidence that asthma is more common in CVID than in XLA, as 31.2% of patients with CVID in the national registry had a diagnosis of asthma compared with 10.3% of those with XLA.[33] In the same study, we found asthma to be the most common chronic pulmonary complication in CVID, but there was no association with age of symptom onset or CVID diagnosis. Like CVID, those with IgAD have an increased likelihood of asthma.[39,40] Even though IgE may contribute to asthma pathology, severe antibody deficiency does not seem to be protective as airway bronchoconstriction in response to allergens can occur in CVID when IgE-mediated allergy testing is negative.[40,41] Although obstructive lung function is often used to diagnose asthma, 1 study found only 9 of 29 patients with CVID with obstructive lung disease to have asthma.[41] Thus, alternative etiologies of obstructive lung disease must be considered in PAD as many cases may be misdiagnosed as asthma.

Little is known regarding the relationship of PAD with COPD. PAD seems to result in more frequent COPD exacerbations and low levels of IgA have been proposed to underlie COPD exacerbation and/or progression.[42–44] Population studies of PAD have not differentiated rates of COPD from that of asthma definitively, but when both forms of obstructive lung disease are considered together they were found in 19% of patients with CVID in 1 study.[45] It is unclear whether risks of smoking are heightened in patients with PAD, but it is a habit that is certainly advisable to halt as in any patient. Thus, although the data are limited, evidence suggests that, like asthma, COPD prevalence and exacerbation rate are increased in PAD.

It is reasonable to postulate that PAD predisposes to respiratory infections that can promote asthma or COPD. Yet, the precise mechanism by which PAD promotes asthma or COPD remains to be conclusively defined. Numerous studies have demonstrated benefit of IRT for asthma or COPD in various types of PAD.[13,46–48] Other than the provision of IRT, management of asthma and COPD in patients with PAD follows standardized diagnostic and treatment guidelines reviewed in detail elsewhere.[49,50] However, the efficacy of specific treatments have not been tested in PAD and it is possible that some agents, most notably immunomodulatory biologics, may have differing efficacy compared with the general population. It should be noted that some patients with PAD may have immune defects contributing to obstructive lung disease that are not fully ameliorated by IRT. Indeed, we found asthma to be associated with lower levels of IgA and IgM in CVID, and these antibody isotypes are not significantly provided by IRT therapy.[33] Considerations regarding asthma and COPD in patients with PAD are highlighted in **Box 2**. Further efforts are needed to better understand asthma and COPD within the unique concerns of PAD.

BRONCHIECTASIS

Patients with PAD are particularly at risk of severe lung infections, with 60% or more of patients with CVID and XLA reporting a history of pneumonia before diagnosis of immune deficiency.[11,12,23,32,51] Bronchiectasis can be a complication of recurrent pneumonia and results from irreversible dilation of the airways due to repeated episodes of inflammatory damage.[23,52] PAD is likely to increase the frequency of pulmonary infections that drive airway inflammation and lead to the fixed changes that define bronchiectasis.[53] Chronic rhinosinusitis was found in nearly half of the 900 patients with bronchiectasis and was significantly associated with antibody deficiency in these subjects from a recent report.[54] Further highlighting the cumulative impact of pulmonary infections, bronchiectasis was associated with history of pneumonia, older age, and diagnostic delay in CVID as well as reduced levels of CD4+ T cells and IgM.[29,55–57]

Patients with less severe forms of PAD, such as IgG subclass deficiency, selective IgA deficiency, and specific antibody deficiency, may also have an increased risk of bronchiectasis.[58–62] Lower levels of IgA and/or IgM are associated with bronchiectasis, highlighting that isotypes other than the IgG replaced by IRT could be important in limiting this chronic lung complication.[63] Indeed, local production of IgA and IgM is

---

Box 2
Considerations regarding asthma and COPD in patients with PAD

- Risk of developing obstructive lung disease seems to be increased by PAD.

- As many cases of pulmonary obstruction in PAD may be misdiagnosed as asthma, it is important to confirm the diagnosis and/or rule out alternatives.

- Other than the provision of IRT when indicated, management of asthma and COPD in patients with PAD follows the standard diagnostic and treatment guidelines.

- No studies have been conducted to determine whether changes in conventional management of asthma or COPD is warranted in PAD, or whether specific biologic therapies have more or less utility for patients with immune deficiency.

thought to contribute significantly to mucosal immunity.[64] Specific genetic defects are also key, as exemplified by the high rate of bronchiectasis occurring in those with gain-of-function mutations of *PI3KD*.[65] Excess mucus production and impaired mucociliary clearance that results from bronchiectasis alters the microbial composition of the airways in a manner that promotes a viscous cycle of pulmonary exacerbations.[66] Antibody deficiency itself also clearly alters the constituency and reduces the diversity of mucosal microbiota.[67,68] Another key factor is time, as bronchiectasis is more common in older patients with CVID and XLA.[29,55] Bronchiectasis emerges and progresses in patients with PAD for numerous reasons that must be better targeted therapeutically to improve patient care (**Box 3**).

Clinical presentation of bronchiectasis typically includes chronic cough with purulent sputum, occasional hemoptysis, and dyspnea. Airflow obstruction is often evident on PFT and diagnosis is typically made by computed tomography (CT) as chest radiographs can be inadequate (**Fig. 1**).[69–71] As further evidence that imaging is critical for diagnosis, a recent European study found that cough was more strongly associated with bronchiectasis on a CT scan than spirometry findings in patients with PAD.[57] Observations that can precede bronchiectasis, such as early bronchial wall thickening, may also be identified by a chest CT scan.[72] The clinical impact of bronchiectasis may be more severe in PAD as these patients seem to have heighted inflammation in the lungs and circulation compared with those without immune deficiency but similar degree of bronchiectasis evident on CT scan.[73] Colonization of the airways with nontuberculous mycobacteria (NTM) or *Pseudomonas aeruginosa* can further worsen disease course in patients with bronchiectasis.[74] Sputum culture to rule out such colonization is often helpful in selection of antibiotics and is of particular importance to limit NTM antimicrobial resistance associated with macrolide single therapy.[75] The key points for the diagnostic algorithm of bronchiectasis is highlighted in **Box 4**.

Upon recognition of the immune deficiency, bronchiectasis course in patients with PAD parallels those developing this pulmonary complication from other causes.[76] Treatment options for bronchiectasis in patients with PAD include IgG replacement with a high goal trough (such as 1000 mg/dL), inhaled corticosteroids, and long-acting β-agonists, extended course macrolide therapy, and pulmonary rehabilitation (**Fig. 2**).[77–80] As previously mentioned, before initiating extended course macrolide therapy, sputum culture is recommended to limit NTM resistance. Macrolide therapy has been studied from 8 weeks to 24 months in those with noncystic fibrosis bronchiectasis, but not specifically PAD. The macrolides studied include azithromycin (typically 250 or 500 mg 3 days a week), clarithromycin, and erythromycin.[80–82] Inhaled antibiotics and mucolytics are other potential therapeutic options for PAD-associated bronchiectasis that have been less frequently used.[83,84] Unfortunately, studies evaluating the efficacy of individual therapies for bronchiectasis in PAD are lacking.

Box 3
Key factors that may increase risk of bronchiectasis in PAD

- History of pneumonia, older age, and diagnostic delay.
- Lower levels of CD4+ T cells, IgA, or IgM.
- Specific genetic defects of the immune system, such as gain-of-function mutations *PI3KD*.
- Alterations in microbial composition of the airways.

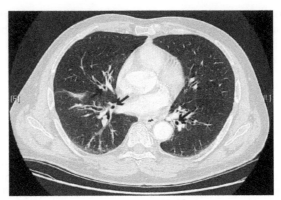

Fig. 1. Bronchial wall thickening (marked by *black arrows*) consistent with bronchiectasis in a patient with PAD.

INTERSTITIAL LUNG DISEASE

The exact prevalence of interstitial lung disease (ILD) in PAD is unclear and varies by immune deficiency. Based on best estimates, ILD occurs in approximately 10% to 20% of patients with CVID.[85] This prevalence may be underestimated as CT findings consistent with ILD (ground glass opacity and/or numerous pulmonary nodules) was noted in 64% of patients with CVID with respiratory symptoms at a tertiary referral center.[55] Interpretation of these CT findings is complicated by the fact that PFT is not always diminished and they may not be indicative of clinically significant ILD.[86,87] ILD seems far less common in other forms of PAD. ILD was absent or exquisitely rare in numerous large studies of X-linked and autosomal recessive hyper IgM syndrome.[88–90] ILD is also very rare in those with congenital agammaglobulinemia, particularly XLA.[32,91–95] We leveraged the expansive USIDNET registry to more closely examine why ILD is more common in CVID than XLA despite both being severe forms of PAD. We found that concurrent autoimmunity and deficiency of T cells were associated with ILD in CVID, immunologic characteristics that occur far less frequently in XLA.[33] Reduction of CD8+ T cells, CD4+ regulatory T cells, and isotype-switched memory B cells, as well as increased serum IgM and CD38+IgM+CD27− transitional B cells have also been associated with presence of ILD or progression in CVID.[96–100] Similarly, ILD has been reported in IgAD patients with autoimmunity and more severe immune defect, such as concurrent IgG subclass deficiency.[4,59,101,102] Thus, alterations in T-cell function, generalized immune dysregulation, greater infection

---

Box 4
Diagnosis of bronchiectasis in PAD

- Clinical presentation includes chronic cough, often with purulent sputum, and dyspnea.
- Airflow obstruction is often evident on PFT.
- CT is usually needed for diagnosis because chest radiographs are frequently inadequate.
- CT can identify precursors of bronchiectasis, such as early bronchial wall thickening.
- Sputum culture can be helpful for selection of antibiotics and identification of colonization with NTM or *Pseudomonas*.

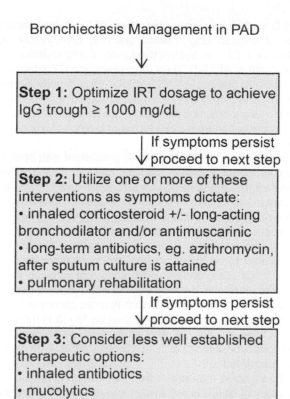

Fig. 2. Proposed algorithm for bronchiectasis management in PAD. IRT, Immunoglobulin replacement therapy.

susceptibility, and/or the presence of pathogenic B cells may be fundamental to the development of ILD in PAD (**Box 5**). Given the heterogeneity of ILD seen in CVID, not all patients should be expected to manifest all these immunologic alterations.

ILD can be challenging to differentiate from other forms of chronic lung disease based on clinical history alone, as the most common presenting symptoms, chronic cough and dyspnea, are nonspecific. Physical examination can be useful, with crackles more indicative of ILD and wheezing more likely to be associated with obstructive disease, such as asthma or COPD. However, physical examination findings can straddle multiple potential diagnoses, as inspiratory ronchi can be heard in

---

Box 5
Immunologic characteristics associated in patients with PAD with ILD

- Greater immune defect as manifested by more profound loss of immunoglobulins, isotype-switched memory B cells, and T cells.
- Deficient or impaired regulatory T cells.
- Increase of serum IgM or IgM + CD38+CD27− transitional B cells.
- Presence of systemic immune dysregulation as demonstrated by history of autoimmunity, lymphadenopathy, and/or splenomegaly.

certain types of ILD as well as some asthmatics. PFT can be useful to differentiate obstructive forms of chronic lung disease (asthma, bronchiectasis, COPD) from restrictive lung disease (ILD). Yet, obstructive forms of lung disease, such as bronchiectasis, can occur together with ILD. Thus, high-resolution CT is frequently vital for the evaluation of chronic lung disease in PAD, with ILD often manifesting as large pulmonary nodules (**Fig. 3**). Lung biopsy can be helpful to confirm a diagnosis of ILD, rule out lymphoma or other malignancy, and perhaps even help guide therapy.[103] The diagnosis of ILD and differentiation from other forms of pulmonary disease requires using various modalities of clinical evaluation.

ILD pathology in patients with PAD is typically consistent with one or more forms of benign pulmonary lymphoproliferation, usually follicular bronchiolitis, lymphocytic interstitial pneumonia (LIP), or nodular lymphoid hyperplasia.[55,97,104] In follicular bronchiolitis, there is benign hyperplasia of lymphoid follicles adjacent to airways (**Fig. 4**A). LIP is considered a progression of this pulmonary lymphoid hyperplasia into the lung interstitium with expansion of alveoli septa (**Fig. 4**B). Nodular lymphoid hyperplasia in the lungs is characterized by lymphoid follicles that are more cleanly demarcated than in LIP and is speculated to be a precursor of mucosal-associated lymphoid tissue (MALT) lymphoma.[104] Of note, patients with CVID are occasionally misdiagnosed with MALT lymphoma when this diagnosis is not adequately differentiated from the benign lymphoproliferative lung pathology that is most common.[105] Granulomatous inflammation and organizing pneumonia may also be found in lungs of patients with PAD together with one of the lymphoproliferative pathologies, and the term granulomatous-lymphocytic interstitial lung disease (GLILD) is frequently used to described the ILD associated with PAD.[106–108] Granulomas and organizing pneumonia are features of LIP, so some may prefer this terminology over GLILD.[109,110] As the multifaceted pathology of GLILD is not always appreciated, it is imperative recognize the spectrum of ILD pathologies found in PAD (**Table 1**).

Perceived similarities with sarcoidosis can present another challenge when evaluating ILD in PAD. In both conditions, granulomatous inflammation can occur inside as well as outside the lungs and pulmonary imaging can look similar at first glance. Sarcoidosis is typically distinguished radiologically by smaller pulmonary nodules that have an apical or perilymphatic distribution, compared with the larger nodules with generalized lung distribution in PAD.[111] When available, biopsies can differentiate the conditions, as PAD ILD typically demonstrates benign lymphoproliferation (eg, follicular bronchiolitis, LIP) that is generally absent in sarcoidosis. Clinical and laboratory features of patients with PAD, such as history of autoimmune cytopenia, nodular

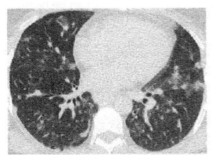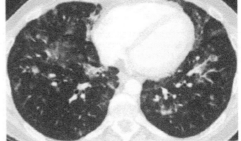

Fig. 3. CT chest imaging from 2 distinct patients with CVID demonstrating large nodules typical of PAD-associated ILD.

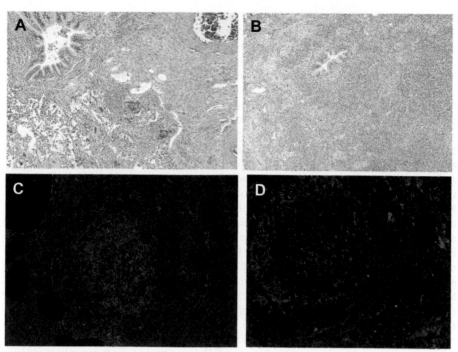

Fig. 4. Immunopathology of CVID ILD. (*A*) Hematoxylin and eosin (H&E) stain demonstrating peribronchial lymphocytic inflammation of follicular bronchiolitis in a patient with CVID. (*B*) H&E stain showing expansion of peribronchial inflammation into lymphocytic interstitial pneumonia (LIP) in a patient with CVID. (*C*) Immunofluorescence demonstrating IgD+ B cells (*green*) In ectopic pulmonary follicles with adjacent IgM^{bright} B cells (*red*) with diamidino-phenylindole (DAPI) (*blue*) nuclear stain. (*D*) IgD+ B cells (*green*) and B-cell activating factor (BAFF) in CVID ILD with DAPI (*blue*) nuclear stain.

Table 1
Types of interstitial lung disease pathology seen in primary antibody deficiency

Pathology	Characteristics
Follicular bronchiolitis	Benign lymphoid hyperplasia bordering the airways
Lymphocytic interstitial pneumonia	Pulmonary lymphoid hyperplasia involving lung interstitium with expansion of alveoli septa. Considered progression of follicular bronchiolitis. Granulomas may be present
Nodular lymphoid hyperplasia	Well-demarcated lymphoid follicles considered a precursor to MALT lymphoma
Non-necrotizing granulomatous inflammation	Inflammation containing circumscribed macrophages lacking a central area of necrosis
Organizing pneumonia	Production of granulation tissue within the alveolar space in response to lung injury. Formerly called bronchiolitis obliterans with organizing pneumonia or BOOP
GLILD	Broadly encompassing term typically implying the presence of granulomatous inflammation together with pulmonary lymphoid hyperplasia and sometimes also organizing pneumonia

regenerative hyperplasia of the liver, recurrent infections, and splenomegaly, as well as antibody deficiency and diminished isotype-switched memory B cells, should raise suspicion of PAD more so than sarcoidosis. Although not in all PAD ILD cases, bronchiectasis is far more suggestive of immune deficiency than sarcoidosis when it is found. Newer tests allowing for rapid identification of patients with severe PAD, such as measurement of serum B-cell maturation antigen, may also prove to be useful.[112] Thus, numerous differences between PAD-associated ILD and sarcoidosis can be exploited to differentiate these chronic lung diseases (**Table 2**).

The pathologic basis of ILD in PAD remains largely unknown. Initial perceptions held that infection drove ILD development. Associations have been made with human herpes virus 8 and Epstein-Barr virus, which have been shown to underlie lymphoproliferation in other patients.[113–117] These viral etiologies have not been identified in the vast majority of cases of PAD ILD, although improved diagnostic approaches, such as next-generation sequencing, may be needed.[118] Bronchiectasis, a frequent complication of PAD, can develop into follicular bronchiolitis, a common form of ILD seen in PAD.[119,120] Although we found a significant association between bronchiectasis and ILD in patients with CVID from USIDNET, there was no association of these complications in our single-center study.[33,55] This discrepancy may be explained by input error in USIDNET, as the registry did not require CT or biopsy confirmation of the pulmonary diagnosis as was required in the single-center study. Alternatively, tertiary referral sites like the single-center study may receive a higher proportion of patients for which the ILD results from systemic immune regulation, due to the multisystem problems that often lead to their referral, whereas at other sites chronic infection may be a key driver of the forms of ILD encountered. As there is heterogeneity among the ILD occurring in PAD, etiologies could vary.[121]

There are numerous lines of evidence that suggest infection is not required for the development of ILD in PAD. Particularly in patients with CVID, ILD frequently occurs in conjunction with lymphoid hyperplasia in other tissues, such as lymph nodes, spleen,

Table 2
Differentiating primary antibody deficiency-associated interstitial lung disease from sarcoidosis

Clinical Feature	PAD-Associated ILD	Sarcoidosis
Low immunoglobulins	+	−
Low isotype-switched memory B cells	+	−
Recurrent infections	+	−
Autoimmune cytopenia, nodular regenerative hyperplasia of the liver, and/or splenomegaly	+	−
Follicular bronchiolitis	+	−
Lymphocytic interstitial pneumonia	+	−
Radiology feature		
Large nodules (>1 cm)	+	−
Small nodules (<1 cm)	−	+
Nodules localized to apical lung zones and perilymphatic regions	−	+
Nodules with generalized distribution within lungs	+	−
Bronchiectasis	+	−

and the mucosal lymphoid tissue of the gastrointestinal tract.[55,96,97,122,123] Thus, the pulmonary lymphoid hyperplasia that characterizes the ILD seen in PAD may reflect systemic immune dysregulation inherent to the patient.[31,124] Along these lines, auto-immunity is more common in patients with CVID with ILD, mirroring the association observed in other immunologic diseases, such as rheumatoid arthritis and Sjögren's syndrome.[73,100,125,126] The importance of intrinsic immune dysregulation is also exemplified by CVID-like disorders with monogenic etiologies. Haploinsufficiency of cytotoxic T lymphocyte-associated protein 4 (CTLA-4) can result in an immune dysregulation syndrome in which PAD is a prominent feature and ILD occurs frequently.[127–129] Autosomal recessive defects of lipopolysaccharide-responsive beige-like anchor protein (LRBA) impair trafficking of CTLA-4 and result in a similar immune dysregulation syndrome in which ILD occurs frequently.[130–132] Autosomal dominant gain-of-function mutations of PI3KD or STAT3 also result in immune dysregulation disorders characterized by antibody deficiency and ILD along with auto-immunity and generalized lymphoproliferation.[133–136] These strong links with intrinsic immune dysregulation provide evidence that infection is not required for ILD in PAD.

A predominant feature of the pulmonary lymphoid hyperplasia seen in CVID ILD are ectopic B-cell follicles that predominantly express IgD along with IgM-producing cells that express markers of plasmablasts and are more numerous in patients with PFT decline (**Fig. 4C**).[98] In addition to showing evidence of active proliferation, these B-cell follicles express markers of germinal centers, a curious finding considering the extensive B-cell maturation defect in many of the affected forms of PAD, such as CVID, and the apparent absence of antibody isotype switching.[137] As both protective and autoreactive immune responses can be generated within ectopic follicles, these lymphoid sites have important roles in both immune protection and pathology.[138] The clinical significance of pathogenic B cells in CVID ILD has been recognized for years and rituximab has been used for treatment as part of either single or combination therapy by numerous groups.[137,139–142] We recently reported the largest study of rituximab for CVID ILD, demonstrating clear efficacy of the intervention over supportive care.[98] ILD recurred after B-cell depletion in about one-third of our subjects in association with increased B-cell activating factor (BAFF) (**Fig. 4D**), which we demonstrated in the same study to help oppose apoptosis of B cells and serve as a potential driver of lymphoid hyperplasia in the lungs of CVID patients. Research efforts are ongoing to enhance our understanding of this potential key mechanism of disease pathogenesis.

The question of when and who to treat for ILD can be challenging. It is clear that pulmonary nodules can wax and wane in patients with PAD and PFT can remain stable for extended periods.[87,98] It is imperative that IgG replacement therapy is optimized in patients with ILD because there may be a subset of patients for which ILD is stabilized by this intervention and patients with CVID with troughs of 1000 mg/dL or greater are less likely to have pulmonary function decline.[87,143] A reasonable option for the next intervention in PAD with mild to moderate ILD symptoms is inhaled corticosteroids, with or without long-acting beta agonists, and/or prophylactic macrolides as these therapies have been shown efficacious in follicular bronchiolitis.[144–146] Systemic corticosteroid treatment may also be efficacious, with the caveats that long-term usage of these agents is frequently associated with adverse effects that outweigh their utility and many cases end up refractory to this intervention.[147]

In addition to the previously mentioned rituximab, a variety of immunomodulators have been used to manage PAD-associated ILD. These include azathioprine, cyclosporine, cyclophosphamide, hydroxychorloquine, methotrexate, and mycophenolate mofetil, individually or used together with rituximab.[139,148] Patients with CVID with prominent granulomatous inflammation may be responsive to tumor necrosis factor antagonists.[149,150] Rituximab offers the advantage of limiting additional immune suppression in patients who already have PAD and are on IRT, as well as having lower risk of adverse effects, such as infection and malignancy, as other immunomodulatory agents.[151,152] In those in which ILD recurs after rituximab, we have found that addition of azathioprine or mycophenolate mofetil is effective in inducing longer remission after B-cell depletion.[98] Given the evidence that BAFF promotes ILD recurrence, BAFF depletive therapies, such as belimumab, may also be useful to prevent recurrence. Patients without prominent pulmonary B-cell follicles may not benefit as much from B-cell–targeted therapy and those with significant fibrosis may not see significant improvement from any type of immunomodulation.

Precision therapy is available for CVID-like diseases with monogenic etiologies. Abatacept can rectify the protein deficiencies of CTLA-4 due to mutations of *CTLA4* or *LRBA*.[153] In another example of treatment tailored to the genetic defect, those

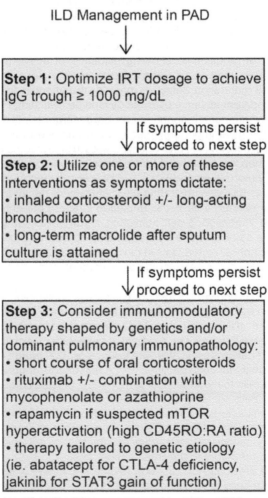

Fig. 5. Proposed algorithm for ILD management in PAD. mTOR, mammalian target of rapamycin.

Box 6
Fundamental diagnostic tools for evaluation of chronic lung disease in PAD

- "Baseline" PFT at PAD diagnosis and then as dictated by symptoms or physician discretion.
- Baseline CT chest at PAD diagnosis and then as dictated by symptoms and/or findings.
- If biopsy is pursued, video-assisted thoracoscopic biopsy is preferred over endobronchial.
- Sputum microbiology is helpful to rule out NTM and *Pseudomonas* colonization.
- In patients with ILD, abrupt increases in serum IgM or circulating B cells post-rituximab could be harbingers of disease progression or recurrence.

---

with gain-of-function mutation of *PI3KD* are responsive to targeted inhibition of phosphoinositide 3-kinase δ with leniolisib.[154] A less precise, but effective, alternative for these forms of PAD with lymphoproliferation is rapamycin, as they each have hyperactivation of the mTOR pathway.[127,136] Rapamycin has shown efficacy in other patients with PAD with GLILD and may have its greatest potential benefit in those with increased ratios of CD45RO+ effector to CD45RA+ naive T cells and/or reduced levels of regulatory T cells.[99] Targeted inhibition of gain-of-function mutations in *STAT3* with jakinibs also may provide benefit for ILD in these patients.[155] In addition to pathologic characteristics, genetic findings can profoundly shape therapeutic options and potential efficacy. Given the monumental risks involved and generally poor results, lung transplant is reserved as a last resort.[156] Bone marrow transplant may improve complications of immune dysregulation in CVID, but the exorbitant mortality rate (upward of 50%) makes this option undesirable until outcomes are improved.[157] Approach to the treatment of ILD in PAD is presented in **Fig. 5**.

SUMMARY

The evaluation of a patient with PAD with suspected chronic lung disease involves several fundamental diagnostic tools (**Box 6**). Imaging and PFT form the basis of any diagnostic work-up and together can help differentiate various forms of lung disease occurring in PAD. Even in those without respiratory symptoms, a "baseline" high-resolution chest CT and PFT seem prudent at the time of diagnosis of PAD to look for evidence of chronic lung disease that may be present before onset of symptoms. These baseline findings can be useful to determine any changes in association with clinical symptoms at a later date. It is usually unnecessary to conduct repeated chest imaging in asymptomatic and uncomplicated patients who are adherent with therapy. ILD is usually present at diagnosis of PAD and does not develop insidiously in those without evidence of lung disease or other complications.[31,55,158] Bronchiectasis may develop over the course of years with minimal symptoms, but the utility of repeated imaging to look for asymptomatic progression is unclear.

Monitoring of pulmonary nodules as per typical guidelines may be controversial in patients with PAD given the increased risk of malignancy in some patients, such as those with CVID. However, in our experience many of these nodules are benign and many wax and wane over time, indicating that aggressively low thresholds to biopsy (and repeated biopsies) may not be necessary. Magnetic resonance imaging offers an option for repeated chest surveillance without radiation exposure and may be a useful for clinicians desiring more frequent monitoring.[159,160] Biopsies are useful to determine the etiology of expanding nodules or potentially guide therapy by the predominant pathology in those with clinical worsening. Video-assisted thoracoscopic surgical biopsy is preferable over endobronchial biopsy to increase tissue yield so that the pulmonary pathology can be more accurately discerned.

PFT is another useful tool for monitoring chronic lung disease. We typically advise PFT every 6 to 12 months in patients with PAD with moderate to severe chronic lung disease, with more frequent testing as symptoms dictate. Notably, diffusion capacity of the lung for carbon monoxide (DLCO) decline may precede changes in other PFT parameters in patients with PAD with ILD, thus evaluations that exclude this measurement may be suboptimal.[87] In patients with PAD with ILD there are other, less validated, tools that can be used to monitor disease progression. We found serum IgM to increase with PFT decline in a subset of patients with CVID with ILD consistent with pulmonary lymphoid hyperplasia.[87,98] Rapid replenishment and/or increase of circulating B cells may be a harbinger of ILD recurrence in patients with PAD after rituximab therapy. However, given the heterogeneity of ILD pathology in patients with PAD, some with minimal presence of B cells, a unifying biomarker for monitoring disease progression in all patients, remains elusive. Efforts remain ongoing to enhance our understanding and improve management of the spectrum of chronic lung diseases affecting patients with PAD.

ACKNOWLEDGMENTS

P.J. Maglione is supported by NIH grant AI137183 and AI151486, a faculty development award from the American Association of Allergy, Asthma and Immunology Foundation, Boston University, and investigator-initiated grants from Horizon and Takeda.

REFERENCES

1. Smith T, Cunningham-Rundles C. Primary B-cell immunodeficiencies. Hum Immunol 2019;80:351–62.
2. Durandy A, Kracker S, Fischer A. Primary antibody deficiencies. Nat Rev Immunol 2013;13:519–33.
3. Cunningham-Rundles C, Maglione PJ. Common variable immunodeficiency. J Allergy Clin Immunol 2012;129:1425–6.e3.
4. Schussler E, Beasley MB, Maglione PJ. Lung disease in primary antibody deficiencies. J Allergy Clin Immunol Pract 2016;4:1039–52.
5. Slade CA, Bosco JJ, Binh Giang T, et al. Delayed diagnosis and complications of predominantly antibody deficiencies in a cohort of Australian adults. Front Immunol 2018;9:694.
6. Wood P. Primary antibody deficiencies: recognition, clinical diagnosis and referral of patients. Clin Med (Lond) 2009;9:595–9.
7. Bonilla FA, Khan DA, Ballas ZK, et al. Practice parameter for the diagnosis and management of primary immunodeficiency. J Allergy Clin Immunol 2015;136:1186–205.e1-78.
8. Gregersen S, Aalokken TM, Mynarek G, et al. Development of pulmonary abnormalities in patients with common variable immunodeficiency: associations with clinical and immunologic factors. Ann Allergy Asthma Immunol 2010;104:503–10.
9. Sweinberg SK, Wodell RA, Grodofsky MP, et al. Retrospective analysis of the incidence of pulmonary disease in hypogammaglobulinemia. J Allergy Clin Immunol 1991;88:96–104.
10. Obregon RG, Lynch DA, Kaske T, et al. Radiologic findings of adult primary immunodeficiency disorders. Contribution of CT. Chest 1994;106:490–5.

11. Busse PJ, Razvi S, Cunningham-Rundles C. Efficacy of intravenous immuno-globulin in the prevention of pneumonia in patients with common variable immu-nodeficiency. J Allergy Clin Immunol 2002;109:1001–4.
12. Orange JS, Grossman WJ, Navickis RJ, et al. Impact of trough IgG on pneu-monia incidence in primary immunodeficiency: a meta-analysis of clinical studies. Clin Immunol 2010;137:21–30.
13. van Kessel DA, Hoffman TW, van Velzen-Blad H, et al. Long-term clinical outcome of antibody replacement therapy in humoral immunodeficient adults with respiratory tract infections. EBioMedicine 2017;18:254–60.
14. Gernez Y, Baker MG, Maglione PJ. Humoral immunodeficiencies: conferred risk of infections and benefits of immunoglobulin replacement therapy. Transfusion 2018;58(Suppl 3):3056–64.
15. Lederman HM, Winkelstein JA. X-linked agammaglobulinemia: an analysis of 96 patients. Medicine (Baltimore) 1985;64:145–56.
16. Hermaszewski RA, Webster AD. Primary hypogammaglobulinaemia: a survey of clinical manifestations and complications. Q J Med 1993;86:31–42.
17. Milito C, Pulvirenti F, Cinetto F, et al. Double-blind, placebo-controlled, random-ized trial on low-dose azithromycin prophylaxis in patients with primary antibody deficiencies. J Allergy Clin Immunol 2019;144:584–93.e7.
18. Kainulainen L, Vuorlnen T, Rantakokko-Jalava K, et al. Recurrent and persistent respiratory tract viral infections in patients with primary hypogammaglobulin-emia. J Allergy Clin Immunol 2010;126:120–6.
19. Jones TPW, Buckland M, Breuer J, et al. Viral infection in primary antibody defi-ciency syndromes. Rev Med Virol 2019;29:e2049.
20. Peltola V, Waris M, Kainulainen L, et al. Virus shedding after human rhinovirus infection in children, adults and patients with hypogammaglobulinaemia. Clin Microbiol Infect 2013;19:E322–7.
21. Chen Y, Stirling RG, Paul E, et al. Longitudinal decline in lung function in patients with primary immunoglobulin deficiencies. J Allergy Clin Immunol 2011;127:1414–7.
22. Resnick ES, Moshier EL, Godbold JH, et al. Morbidity and mortality in common variable immune deficiency over 4 decades. Blood 2012;119:1650–7.
23. Notarangelo LD, Plebani A, Mazzolari E, et al. Genetic causes of bronchiectasis: primary immune deficiencies and the lung. Respiration 2007;74:264–75.
24. Buckley RH. Pulmonary complications of primary immunodeficiencies. Paediatr Respir Rev 2004;5(Suppl A):S225–33.
25. Eijkhout HW, van Der Meer JW, Kallenberg CG, et al. The effect of two different dosages of intravenous immunoglobulin on the incidence of recurrent infections in patients with primary hypogammaglobulinemia. A randomized, double-blind, multicenter crossover trial. Ann Intern Med 2001;135:165–74.
26. Stiehm ER, Chin TW, Haas A, et al. Infectious complications of the primary im-munodeficiencies. Clin Immunol Immunopathol 1986;40:69–86.
27. Janeway CA, Rosen FS. The gamma globulins. IV. Therapeutic uses of gamma globulin. N Engl J Med 1966;275:826–31.
28. Stubbs A, Bangs C, Shillitoe B, et al. Bronchiectasis and deteriorating lung func-tion in agammaglobulinaemia despite immunoglobulin replacement therapy. Clin Exp Immunol 2018;191:212–9.
29. Quinti I, Soresina A, Guerra A, et al. Effectiveness of immunoglobulin replace-ment therapy on clinical outcome in patients with primary antibody deficiencies: results from a multicenter prospective cohort study. J Clin Immunol 2011;31:315–22.

30. Plebani A, Soresina A, Rondelli R, et al. Clinical, immunological, and molecular analysis in a large cohort of patients with X-linked agammaglobulinemia: an Italian multicenter study. Clin Immunol 2002;104:221–30.
31. Maglione PJ. Autoimmune and lymphoproliferative complications of common variable immunodeficiency. Curr Allergy Asthma Rep 2016;16:19.
32. Aghamohammadi A, Allahverdi A, Abolhassani H, et al. Comparison of pulmonary diseases in common variable immunodeficiency and X-linked agammaglobulinaemia. Respirology 2010;15:289–95.
33. Weinberger T, Fuleihan R, Cunningham-Rundles C, et al. Factors beyond lack of antibody govern pulmonary complications in primary antibody deficiency. J Clin Immunol 2019;39:440–7.
34. Durandy A, Peron S, Fischer A. Hyper-IgM syndromes. Curr Opin Rheumatol 2006;18:369–76.
35. Jolles S, Sanchez-Ramon S, Quinti I, et al. Screening protocols to monitor respiratory status in primary immunodeficiency disease: findings from a European survey and subclinical infection working group. Clin Exp Immunol 2017;190: 226–34.
36. Reisi M, Azizi G, Kiaee F, et al. Evaluation of pulmonary complications in patients with primary immunodeficiency disorders. Eur Ann Allergy Clin Immunol 2017; 49:122–8.
37. Milota T, Bloomfield M, Parackova Z, et al. Bronchial asthma and bronchial hyperresponsiveness and their characteristics in patients with common variable immunodeficiency. Int Arch Allergy Immunol 2019;178:192–200.
38. Farmer JR, Ong MS, Barmettler S, et al. Common variable immunodeficiency non-infectious disease endotypes redefined using unbiased network clustering in large electronic datasets. Front Immunol 2017;8:1740.
39. Ozcan C, Metin A, Erkocoglu M, et al. Bronchial hyperreactivity in children with antibody deficiencies. Allergol Immunopathol (Madr) 2015;43:57–61.
40. Urm SH, Yun HD, Fenta YA, et al. Asthma and risk of selective IgA deficiency or common variable immunodeficiency: a population-based case-control study. Mayo Clin Proc 2013;88:813–21.
41. Agondi RC, Barros MT, Rizzo LV, et al. Allergic asthma in patients with common variable immunodeficiency. Allergy 2010;65:510–5.
42. McCullagh BN, Comellas AP, Ballas ZK, et al. Antibody deficiency in patients with frequent exacerbations of chronic obstructive pulmonary disease (COPD). PLoS One 2017;12:e0172437.
43. Polosukhin VV, Richmond BW, Du RH, et al. Secretory IgA deficiency in individual small airways is associated with persistent inflammation and remodeling. Am J Respir Crit Care Med 2017;195:1010–21.
44. Putcha N, Paul GG, Azar A, et al. Lower serum IgA is associated with COPD exacerbation risk in SPIROMICS. PLoS One 2018;13:e0194924.
45. Maarschalk-Ellerbroek LJ, de Jong PA, van Montfrans JM, et al. CT screening for pulmonary pathology in common variable immunodeficiency disorders and the correlation with clinical and immunological parameters. J Clin Immunol 2014;34: 642–54.
46. Roifman CM, Gelfand EW. Replacement therapy with high dose intravenous gamma-globulin improves chronic sinopulmonary disease in patients with hypogammaglobulinemia. Pediatr Infect Dis J 1988;7:S92–6.
47. Tiotiu A, Salvator H, Jaussaud R, et al. Efficacy of immunoglobulin replacement therapy and azithromycin in severe asthma with antibody deficiency. Allergol Int 2020;69(2):215–22.

48. Kim JH, Ye YM, Ban GY, et al. Effects of immunoglobulin replacement on asthma exacerbation in adult asthmatics with IgG subclass deficiency. Allergy Asthma Immunol Res 2017;9:526–33.
49. Riley CM, Sciurba FC. Diagnosis and outpatient management of chronic obstructive pulmonary disease: a review. JAMA 2019;321:786–97.
50. Wu TD, Brigham EP, McCormack MC. Asthma in the primary care setting. Med Clin North Am 2019;103:435–52.
51. Winkelstein JA, Marino MC, Lederman HM, et al. X-linked agammaglobulinemia: report on a United States registry of 201 patients. Medicine (Baltimore) 2006;85: 193–202.
52. Barker AF. Bronchiectasis. N Engl J Med 2002;346:1383–93.
53. Cole PJ. Inflammation: a two-edged sword—the model of bronchiectasis. Eur J Respir Dis Suppl 1986;147:6–15.
54. Somani SN, Kwah JH, Yeh C, et al. Prevalence and characterization of chronic rhinosinusitis in patients with non-cystic fibrosis bronchiectasis at a tertiary care center in the United States. Int Forum Allergy Rhinol 2019;9:1424–9.
55. Maglione PJ, Overbey JR, Radigan L, et al. Pulmonary radiologic findings in common variable immunodeficiency: clinical and immunological correlations. Ann Allergy Asthma Immunol 2014;113:452–9.
56. Gathmann B, Mahlaoui N, Gerard L, et al. Clinical picture and treatment of 2212 patients with common variable immunodeficiency. J Allergy Clin Immunol 2014; 134:116–26.
57. Schutz K, Alecsandru D, Grimbacher B, et al. Imaging of bronchial pathology in antibody deficiency: data from the European Chest CT Group. J Clin Immunol 2019;39:45–54.
58. Aghamohammadi A, Cheraghi T, Gharagozlou M, et al. IgA deficiency: correlation between clinical and immunological phenotypes. J Clin Immunol 2009;29: 130–6.
59. Bjorkander J, Bake B, Oxelius VA, et al. Impaired lung function in patients with IgA deficiency and low levels of IgG2 or IgG3. N Engl J Med 1985;313:720–4.
60. Stanley PJ, Corbo G, Cole PJ. Serum IgG subclasses in chronic and recurrent respiratory infections. Clin Exp Immunol 1984;58:703–8.
61. De Gracia J, Rodrigo MJ, Morell F, et al. IgG subclass deficiencies associated with bronchiectasis. Am J Respir Crit Care Med 1996;153:650–5.
62. van Kessel DA, van Velzen-Blad H, van den Bosch JM, et al. Impaired pneumococcal antibody response in bronchiectasis of unknown aetiology. Eur Respir J 2005;25:482–9.
63. Hodkinson JP, Bangs C, Wartenberg-Demand A, et al. Low IgA and IgM is associated with a higher prevalence of bronchiectasis in primary antibody deficiency. J Clin Immunol 2017;37:329–31.
64. Langereis JD, van der Flier M, de Jonge MI. Limited innovations after more than 65 years of immunoglobulin replacement therapy: potential of IgA- and IgM-enriched formulations to prevent bacterial respiratory tract infections. Front Immunol 2018;9:1925.
65. Angulo I, Vadas O, Garcon F, et al. Phosphoinositide 3-kinase delta gene mutation predisposes to respiratory infection and airway damage. Science 2013;342: 866–71.
66. Pereira AC, Kokron CM, Romagnolo BM, et al. Analysis of the sputum and inflammatory alterations of the airways in patients with common variable immunodeficiency and bronchiectasis. Clinics (Sao Paulo) 2009;64:1155–60.

67. Jorgensen SF, Troseid M, Kummen M, et al. Altered gut microbiota profile in common variable immunodeficiency associates with levels of lipopolysaccharide and markers of systemic immune activation. Mucosal Immunol 2016;9: 1455–65.

68. Fadlallah J, El Kafsi H, Sterlin D, et al. Microbial ecology perturbation in human IgA deficiency. Sci Transl Med 2018;10 [pii:eaan1217].

69. King PT, Holdsworth SR, Freezer NJ, et al. Outcome in adult bronchiectasis. COPD 2005;2:27–34.

70. Twiss J, Stewart AW, Byrnes CA. Longitudinal pulmonary function of childhood bronchiectasis and comparison with cystic fibrosis. Thorax 2006;61:414–8.

71. Martinez-Garcia MA, Soler-Cataluna JJ, Perpina-Tordera M, et al. Factors associated with lung function decline in adult patients with stable non-cystic fibrosis bronchiectasis. Chest 2007;132:1565–72.

72. Hampson FA, Chandra A, Screaton NJ, et al. Respiratory disease in common variable immunodeficiency and other primary immunodeficiency disorders. Clin Radiol 2012;67:587–95.

73. Hurst JR, Workman S, Garcha DS, et al. Activity, severity and impact of respiratory disease in primary antibody deficiency syndromes. J Clin Immunol 2014;34: 68–75.

74. Griffith DE, Aksamit TR. Bronchiectasis and nontuberculous mycobacterial disease. Clin Chest Med 2012;33:283–95.

75. Kipourou M, Manika K, Papavasileiou A, et al. Immunomodulatory effect of macrolides: at what cost? Respir Med Case Rep 2016;17:44–6.

76. Goussault H, Salvator H, Catherinot E, et al. Primary immunodeficiency-related bronchiectasis in adults: comparison with bronchiectasis of other etiologies in a French reference center. Respir Res 2019;20:275.

77. Chalmers JD, Aliberti S, Blasi F. Management of bronchiectasis in adults. Eur Respir J 2015;45:1446–62.

78. Bonilla FA, Bernstein IL, Khan DA, et al. Practice parameter for the diagnosis and management of primary immunodeficiency. Ann Allergy Asthma Immunol 2005;94:S1–63.

79. Welsh EJ, Evans DJ, Fowler SJ, et al. Interventions for bronchiectasis: an overview of Cochrane systematic reviews. Cochrane Database Syst Rev 2015;(7):CD010337.

80. Altenburg J, de Graaff CS, Stienstra Y, et al. Effect of azithromycin maintenance treatment on infectious exacerbations among patients with non-cystic fibrosis bronchiectasis: the BAT randomized controlled trial. JAMA 2013;309:1251–9.

81. Wong C, Jayaram L, Karalus N, et al. Azithromycin for prevention of exacerbations in non-cystic fibrosis bronchiectasis (EMBRACE): a randomised, double-blind, placebo-controlled trial. Lancet 2012;380:660–7.

82. Fan LC, Lu HW, Wei P, et al. Effects of long-term use of macrolides in patients with non-cystic fibrosis bronchiectasis: a meta-analysis of randomized controlled trials. BMC Infect Dis 2015;15:160.

83. Tay GT, Reid DW, Bell SC. Inhaled antibiotics in cystic fibrosis (CF) and non-CF bronchiectasis. Semin Respir Crit Care Med 2015;36:267–86.

84. Mall MA, Danahay H, Boucher RC. Emerging concepts and therapies for mucoobstructive lung disease. Ann Am Thorac Soc 2018;15:S216.

85. Verma N, Grimbacher B, Hurst JR. Lung disease in primary antibody deficiency. Lancet Respir Med 2015;3:651–60.

86. Kainulainen L, Varpula M, Liippo K, et al. Pulmonary abnormalities in patients with primary hypogammaglobulinemia. J Allergy Clin Immunol 1999;104: 1031–6.

87. Maglione PJ, Overbey JR, Cunningham-Rundles C. Progression of common variable immunodeficiency interstitial lung disease accompanies distinct pulmonary and laboratory findings. J Allergy Clin Immunol Pract 2015;3:941–50.

88. Winkelstein JA, Marino MC, Ochs H, et al. The X-linked hyper-IgM syndrome: clinical and immunologic features of 79 patients. Medicine (Baltimore) 2003; 82:373–84.

89. Quartier P, Bustamante J, Sanal O, et al. Clinical, immunologic and genetic analysis of 29 patients with autosomal recessive hyper-IgM syndrome due to activation-induced cytidine deaminase deficiency. Clin Immunol 2004;110:22–9.

90. Cabral-Marques O, Klaver S, Schimke LF, et al. First report of the Hyper-IgM syndrome Registry of the Latin American Society for Immunodeficiencies: novel mutations, unique infections, and outcomes. J Clin Immunol 2014;34:146–56.

91. Costa-Carvalho BT, Wandalsen GF, Pulici G, et al. Pulmonary complications in patients with antibody deficiency. Allergol Immunopathol (Madr) 2011;39: 128–32.

92. Toth B, Volokha A, Mihas A, et al. Genetic and demographic features of X-linked agammaglobulinemia in Eastern and Central Europe: a cohort study. Mol Immunol 2009;46:2140–6.

93. Lee PP, Chen TX, Jiang LP, et al. Clinical characteristics and genotype-phenotype correlation in 62 patients with X-linked agammaglobulinemia. J Clin Immunol 2010;30:121–31.

94. Aadam Z, Kechout N, Barakat A, et al. X-Linked agammagobulinemia in a large series of North African patients: frequency, clinical features and novel BTK mutations. J Clin Immunol 2016;36:187–94.

95. Garcia-Garcia E, Staines-Boone AT, Vargas-Hernandez A, et al. Clinical and mutational features of X-linked agammaglobulinemia in Mexico. Clin Immunol 2016;165:38–44.

96. Chapel H, Lucas M, Lee M, et al. Common variable immunodeficiency disorders: division into distinct clinical phenotypes. Blood 2008;112:277–86.

97. Bates CA, Ellison MC, Lynch DA, et al. Granulomatous-lymphocytic lung disease shortens survival in common variable immunodeficiency. J Allergy Clin Immunol 2004;114:415–21.

98. Maglione PJ, Gyimesi G, Cols M, et al. BAFF-driven B cell hyperplasia underlies lung disease in common variable immunodeficiency. JCI Insight 2019;4 [pii: 122728].

99. Deya-Martinez A, Esteve-Sole A, Velez-Tirado N, et al. Sirolimus as an alternative treatment in patients with granulomatous-lymphocytic lung disease and humoral immunodeficiency with impaired regulatory T cells. Pediatr Allergy Immunol 2018;29:425–32.

100. Wehr C, Kivioja T, Schmitt C, et al. The EUROclass trial: defining subgroups in common variable immunodeficiency. Blood 2008;111:77–85.

101. Roca B, Ferran G, Simon E, et al. Lymphoid hyperplasia of the lung and Evans' syndrome in IgA deficiency. Am J Med 1999;106:121–2.

102. Ozkan H, Atlihan F, Genel F, et al. IgA and/or IgG subclass deficiency in children with recurrent respiratory infections and its relationship with chronic pulmonary damage. J Investig Allergol Clin Immunol 2005;15:69–74.

103. Reichenberger F, Wyser C, Gonon M, et al. Pulmonary mucosa-associated lymphoid tissue lymphoma in a patient with common variable immunodeficiency syndrome. Respiration 2001;68:109–12.

104. Carrillo J, Restrepo CS, Rosado de Christenson M, et al. Lymphoproliferative lung disorders: a radiologic-pathologic overview. Part I: reactive disorders. Semin Ultrasound CT MR 2013;34:525–34.

105. da Silva SP, Resnick E, Lucas M, et al. Lymphoid proliferations of indeterminate malignant potential arising in adults with common variable immunodeficiency disorders: unusual case studies and immunohistological review in the light of possible causative events. J Clin Immunol 2011;31:784–91.

106. Ardeniz O, Cunningham-Rundles C. Granulomatous disease in common variable immunodeficiency. Clin Immunol 2009;133:198–207.

107. Roberton BJ, Hansell DM. Organizing pneumonia: a kaleidoscope of concepts and morphologies. Eur Radiol 2011;21:2244–54.

108. Rao N, Mackinnon AC, Routes JM. Granulomatous and lymphocytic interstitial lung disease: a spectrum of pulmonary histopathologic lesions in common variable immunodeficiency—histologic and immunohistochemical analyses of 16 cases. Hum Pathol 2015;46:1306–14.

109. Tian X, Yi ES, Ryu JH. Lymphocytic interstitial pneumonia and other benign lymphoid disorders. Semin Respir Crit Care Med 2012;33:450–61.

110. Guinee DG Jr. Update on nonneoplastic pulmonary lymphoproliferative disorders and related entities. Arch Pathol Lab Med 2010;134:691–701.

111. Verbsky JW, Routes JM. Sarcoidosis and common variable immunodeficiency: similarities and differences. Semin Respir Crit Care Med 2014;35:330–5.

112. Maglione PJ, Ko HM, Tokuyama M, et al. Serum B-cell maturation antigen (BCMA) levels differentiate primary antibody deficiencies. J Allergy Clin Immunol Pract 2020;8(1):283–91.e1.

113. Wheat WH, Cool CD, Morimoto Y, et al. Possible role of human herpesvirus 8 in the lymphoproliferative disorders in common variable immunodeficiency. J Exp Med 2005;202:479–84.

114. Bailey MD, Mitchell GL, Dhaliwal DK, et al. Patient satisfaction and visual symptoms after laser in situ keratomileusis. Ophthalmology 2003;110:1371–8.

115. Barbera JA, Hayashi S, Hegele RG, et al. Detection of Epstein-Barr virus in lymphocytic interstitial pneumonia by in situ hybridization. Am Rev Respir Dis 1992;145:940–6.

116. San-Juan R, Comoli P, Caillard S, et al. Epstein-Barr virus-related post-transplant lymphoproliferative disorder in solid organ transplant recipients. Clin Microbiol Infect 2014;20(Suppl 7):109–18.

117. Unger S, Seidl M, Schmitt-Graeff A, et al. Ill-defined germinal centers and severely reduced plasma cells are histological hallmarks of lymphadenopathy in patients with common variable immunodeficiency. J Clin Immunol 2014;34:615–26.

118. Young BA, Hanson KE, Gomez CA. Molecular diagnostic advances in transplant infectious diseases. Curr Infect Dis Rep 2019;21:52.

119. Ryu JH. Classification and approach to bronchiolar diseases. Curr Opin Pulm Med 2006;12:145–51.

120. Wakamatsu K, Nagata N, Taguchi K, et al. A case of follicular bronchiolitis as the histological counterpart to nodular opacities in bronchiectatic *Mycobacterium avium* complex disease. Case Rep Pulmonol 2012;2012:214601.

121. Patel S, Anzilotti C, Lucas M, et al. Interstitial lung disease in patients with common variable immunodeficiency disorders: several different pathologies? Clin Exp Immunol 2019;198:212–23.

122. Torigian DA, LaRosa DF, Levinson AI, et al. Granulomatous-lymphocytic interstitial lung disease associated with common variable immunodeficiency: CT findings. J Thorac Imaging 2008;23:162–9.

123. Bondioni MP, Soresina A, Lougaris V, et al. Common variable immunodeficiency: computed tomography evaluation of bronchopulmonary changes including nodular lesions in 40 patients. Correlation with clinical and immunological data. J Comput Assist Tomogr 2010;34:395–401.

124. Allenspach E, Torgerson TR. Autoimmunity and primary immunodeficiency disorders. J Clin Immunol 2016;36(Suppl 1):57–67.

125. Bendstrup E, Moller J, Kronborg-White S, et al. Interstitial lung disease in rheumatoid arthritis remains a challenge for clinicians. J Clin Med 2019;8 [pii:E2038].

126. Gupta S, Ferrada MA, Hasni SA. Pulmonary manifestations of primary Sjogren's syndrome: underlying immunological mechanisms, clinical presentation, and management. Front Immunol 2019;10:1327.

127. Kuehn HS, Ouyang W, Lo B, et al. Immune dysregulation in human subjects with heterozygous germline mutations in CTLA4. Science 2014;345:1623–7.

128. Schubert D, Bode C, Kenefeck R, et al. Autosomal dominant immune dysregulation syndrome in humans with CTLA4 mutations. Nat Med 2014;20:1410–6.

129. Schwab C, Gabrysch A, Olbrich P, et al. Phenotype, penetrance, and treatment of 133 cytotoxic T-lymphocyte antigen 4-insufficient subjects. J Allergy Clin Immunol 2018;142:1932–46.

130. Gamez-Diaz L, August D, Stepensky P, et al. The extended phenotype of LPS-responsive beige-like anchor protein (LRBA) deficiency. J Allergy Clin Immunol 2016;137:223–30.

131. Habibi S, Zaki-Dizaji M, Rafiemanesh H, et al. Clinical, immunologic, and molecular spectrum of patients with LPS-responsive beige-like anchor protein deficiency: a systematic review. J Allergy Clin Immunol Pract 2019;7:2379–86.e5.

132. Cagdas D, Halacli SO, Tan C, et al. A spectrum of clinical findings from ALPS to CVID: several novel LRBA defects. J Clin Immunol 2019;39:726–38.

133. Milner JD, Vogel TP, Forbes L, et al. Early-onset lymphoproliferation and autoimmunity caused by germline STAT3 gain-of-function mutations. Blood 2015;125:591–9.

134. Flanagan SE, Haapaniemi E, Russell MA, et al. Activating germline mutations in STAT3 cause early-onset multi-organ autoimmune disease. Nat Genet 2014;46:812–4.

135. Haapaniemi EM, Kaustio M, Rajala HL, et al. Autoimmunity, hypogammaglobulinemia, lymphoproliferation, and mycobacterial disease in patients with activating mutations in STAT3. Blood 2015;125:639–48.

136. Lucas CL, Kuehn HS, Zhao F, et al. Dominant-activating germline mutations in the gene encoding the PI(3)K catalytic subunit p110delta result in T cell senescence and human immunodeficiency. Nat Immunol 2014;15:88–97.

137. Maglione PJ, Ko HM, Beasley MB, et al. Tertiary lymphoid neogenesis is a component of pulmonary lymphoid hyperplasia in patients with common variable immunodeficiency. J Allergy Clin Immunol 2014;133:535–42.

138. Jones GW, Jones SA. Ectopic lymphoid follicles: inducible centres for generating antigen-specific immune responses within tissues. Immunology 2016;147:141–51.

139. Boursiquot JN, Gerard L, Malphettes M, et al. Granulomatous disease in CVID: retrospective analysis of clinical characteristics and treatment efficacy in a cohort of 59 patients. J Clin Immunol 2013;33:84–95.

140. Chase NM, Verbsky JW, Hintermeyer MK, et al. Use of combination chemotherapy for treatment of granulomatous and lymphocytic interstitial lung disease (GLILD) in patients with common variable immunodeficiency (CVID). J Clin Immunol 2013;33:30–9.

141. Jolles S, Carne E, Brouns M, et al. FDG PET-CT imaging of therapeutic response in granulomatous lymphocytic interstitial lung disease (GLILD) in common variable immunodeficiency (CVID). Clin Exp Immunol 2017;187:138–45.

142. Zdziarski P, Gamian A. Lymphoid interstitial pneumonia in common variable immune deficiency—case report with disease monitoring in various therapeutic options: pleiotropic effects of rituximab regimens. Front Pharmacol 2018;9:1559.

143. Arish N, Eldor R, Fellig Y, et al. Lymphocytic interstitial pneumonia associated with common variable immunodeficiency resolved with intravenous immunoglobulins. Thorax 2006;61:1096–7.

144. Hayakawa H, Sato A, Imokawa S, et al. Bronchiolar disease in rheumatoid arthritis. Am J Respir Crit Care Med 1996;154:1531–6.

145. Ryu JH, Myers JL, Swensen SJ. Bronchiolar disorders. Am J Respir Crit Care Med 2003;168:1277–92.

146. Aerni MR, Vassallo R, Myers JL, et al. Follicular bronchiolitis in surgical lung biopsies: clinical implications in 12 patients. Respir Med 2008;102:307–12.

147. Kohler PF, Cook RD, Brown WR, et al. Common variable hypogammaglobulinemia with T-cell nodular lymphoid interstitial pneumonitis and B-cell nodular lymphoid hyperplasia: different lymphocyte populations with a similar response to prednisone therapy. J Allergy Clin Immunol 1982;70:299–305.

148. Davies CW, Juniper MC, Gray W, et al. Lymphoid interstitial pneumonitis associated with common variable hypogammaglobulinaemia treated with cyclosporin A. Thorax 2000;55:88–90.

149. Thatayatikom A, Thatayatikom S, White AJ. Infliximab treatment for severe granulomatous disease in common variable immunodeficiency: a case report and review of the literature. Ann Allergy Asthma Immunol 2005;95:293–300.

150. Franxman TJ, Howe LE, Baker JR Jr. Infliximab for treatment of granulomatous disease in patients with common variable immunodeficiency. J Clin Immunol 2014;34:820–7.

151. Chien SH, Liu CJ, Hong YC, et al. Use of azathioprine for graft-vs-host disease is the major risk for development of secondary malignancies after haematopoietic stem cell transplantation: a nationwide population-based study. Br J Cancer 2015;112:177–84.

152. Gobert D, Bussel JB, Cunningham-Rundles C, et al. Efficacy and safety of rituximab in common variable immunodeficiency-associated immune cytopenias: a retrospective multicentre study on 33 patients. Br J Haematol 2011;155:498–508.

153. Lo B, Zhang K, Lu W, et al. Autoimmune Disease. Patients with LRBA deficiency show CTLA4 loss and immune dysregulation responsive to abatacept therapy. Science 2015;349:436–40.

154. Rao VK, Webster S, Dalm V, et al. Effective "activated PI3Kdelta syndrome"-targeted therapy with the PI3Kdelta inhibitor leniolisib. Blood 2017;130:2307–16.

155. Forbes LR, Vogel TP, Cooper MA, et al. Jakinibs for the treatment of immune dysregulation in patients with gain-of-function signal transducer and activator

of transcription 1 (STAT1) or STAT3 mutations. J Allergy Clin Immunol 2018;142: 1665–9.

156. Burton CM, Milman N, Andersen CB, et al. Common variable immune deficiency and lung transplantation. Scand J Infect Dis 2007;39:362–7.

157. Wehr C, Gennery AR, Lindemans C, et al. Multicenter experience in hematopoietic stem cell transplantation for serious complications of common variable immunodeficiency. J Allergy Clin Immunol 2015;135:988–97.e6.

158. Prasse A, Kayser G, Warnatz K. Common variable immunodeficiency-associated granulomatous and interstitial lung disease. Curr Opin Pulm Med 2013;19:503–9.

159. Milito C, Pulvirenti F, Serra G, et al. Lung magnetic resonance imaging with diffusion weighted imaging provides regional structural as well as functional information without radiation exposure in primary antibody deficiencies. J Clin Immunol 2015;35:491–500.

160. Arslan S, Poyraz N, Ucar R, et al. Magnetic resonance imaging may be a valuable radiation-free technique for lung pathologies in patients with primary immunodeficiency. J Clin Immunol 2016;36:66–72.

IKAROS Family Zinc Finger 1– Associated Diseases in Primary Immunodeficiency Patients

Cristiane J. Nunes-Santos, MD, Hye Sun Kuehn, PhD,
Sergio D. Rosenzweig, MD, PhD*

KEYWORDS

- IKAROS • Immunodeficiency • Antibody deficiency
- Common variable immunodeficiency • Combined immunodeficiency
- Haploinsufficiency • Dominant negative • Gene dosage

KEY POINTS

- Heterozygous germline mutations in IKAROS family zinc finger 1 (IKZF1) DNA binding domain cause immunodeficiency through at least 2 different mechanisms.
- Haploinsufficiency mutations cause a common variable immune deficiency–like phenotype with a B-cell deficiency, infections, and also increased risk of autoimmunity/immune dysregulation and B-cell acute lymphoblastic leukemia; penetrance does not seem to be complete.
- Dominant negative mutations cause a fully penetrant early-onset combined immunodeficiency with T-cell, B-cell, and myeloid cell defects, increased susceptibility to pneumocystis pneumonia among other microbes, and T-cell acute lymphoblastic leukemia.

INTRODUCTION

IKAROS family zinc finger 1 (IKZF1 or IKAROS) is a hematopoietic zinc finger (ZF) DNA-binding transcription factor that acts as a critical regulator at multiple stages of lymphocyte differentiation, from early multipotent precursors to mature effector cells.[1–3] Regulatory functions in myeloid differentiation have also been ascribed for IKAROS.[4] Knowledge of IKAROS involvement in human disease was initially limited to its tumor suppressive activity, because somatic mutations in *IKZF1* are frequently observed in B-cell progenitor acute lymphoblastic leukemia (ALL), conferring a poor prognosis.[5,6] More recently, a large screening of presumed sporadic

Immunology Service, Department of Laboratory Medicine, National Institutes of Health (NIH) Clinical Center, 10 Center Drive, Building 10, Room 2C410F, Bethesda, MD 20892, USA
* Corresponding author.
E-mail address: srosenzweig@cc.nih.gov

Immunol Allergy Clin N Am 40 (2020) 461–470
https://doi.org/10.1016/j.iac.2020.04.004
0889-8561/20/Published by Elsevier Inc.

cases of B-cell ALL (B-ALL) in childhood identified germline heterozygous mutations in *IKZF1* in 0.9% of patients.[7]

In 2012, Goldman and colleagues[8] described a germline heterozygous allelic variant in *IKZF1* (p.Y210C) leading to immunodeficiency in an infant born with congenital pancytopenia and selective lymphopenia characterized by absence of B and natural killer cells with normal numbers of T cells. In 2016, Kuehn and colleagues,[9] studying 6 probands with common variable immunodeficiency (CVID) and decreased numbers of B cells, identified 6 additional germline heterozygous mutations in *IKZF1* in 29 individuals from 6 families. Several reports followed these 2 initial descriptions and, to date, 22 germline heterozygous allelic variants in *IKZF1* have been reported in the setting of primary immunodeficiency (PID)[8-19] (**Fig. 1A**).

IKAROS belongs to the ZF family of proteins, which also includes Helios/IKZF2, Aiolos/IKZF3, Eos/IKZF4, and Pegasus/IKZF5. All of them share a similar structure characterized by the presence of 2 sets of highly conserved C_2H_2-type ZF motifs. The ZFs located N-terminal to these proteins mediate binding to specific DNA sequences located throughout the genome. The second set of ZFs are located C-terminal and enable the protein-to-protein IKAROS family members interaction as homodimers (eg, IKZF1/IKZF1) or heterodimers (eg, IKZF1/IKZF2). Several IKAROS family members undergo alternative splicing; for example, IKZF1 has at least 17

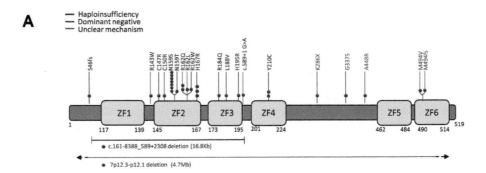

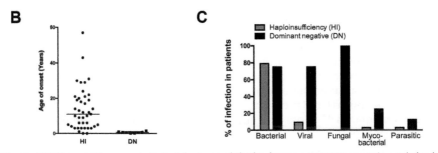

Fig. 1. *IKZF1* mutations and clinical features. (*A*) The human IKAROS protein and the location of mutations. The numbers represent the amino acid location based on *IKZF1* transcript variant 1 (NM_006060). Different molecular mechanisms of *IKZF1* mutations are shown in blue (haploinsufficiency [HI]) and red (dominant negative [DN]). Red circles indicate the number of families carrying the same mutation. (*B*) Age of onset of clinical manifestations in patients with *IKZF1* mutations. Horizontal bars represent median values. (*C*) Infectious agents among symptomatic cases of IKAROS-associated primary immunodeficiency by mechanism of action.

isoforms, adding to the function complexity of these transcription factors (reviewed in Ref.[4,20]).

The main isoform of IKAROS (isoform 1) consists of an N-terminal DNA-binding domain (DBD) comprising 4 ZFs (ZF1–ZF4) and a C-terminal dimerization domain (DD), where 2 more ZFs are located (ZF5 and ZF6). Reported *IKZF1* variants associated with immunodeficiency primarily cluster around the DBD, mostly affecting critical to DNA binding ZF2 and ZF3 (see **Fig. 1A**). Variants located between the DBD and DD (ie, p.K286X, p.G337S, and p.A448R), or directly affecting the DD (p.M494V and p. M494fsX86), have also been reported in patients with CVID.[17] Among these variants, p.K286X and p.M494fsX86 are highly likely to primarily affect IKAROS dimerization and secondarily affect DNA binding or pericentromeric targeting. However, because the pathophysiology of these variants has not yet been completely elucidated, this article focusses on variants with a proven defect on IKAROS-dependent functions (DNA binding and pericentromeric targeting), or directly affecting protein expression.

IKAROS protein expression in lymphocytes was not affected by single amino acid mutants but was reduced to approximately half in patients carrying large deletions or a frameshift mutation leading to an early stop codon (ie, 4.7-Mb deletion and S46AfsX14).[9,12] However, regardless of normal protein expression in patients with missense mutations, in vitro functional assessment revealed that all mutants behaved in a loss-of-function manner, shown by their inability to bind target DNA sequences and to localize to pericentromeric heterochromatin (PC-HC).[8–13,15–17]

Mutants are categorized in 2 groups depending on (1) how they affect the DNA binding to PC-HC, and (2) their effect on the wild-type (WT) allele: heterozygous haploinsufficiency (HI) mutations do not bind target DNA on PC-HC per se, and do not affect the function of the WT allele; in contrast, heterozygous dominant negative (DN) mutations do not bind target DNA on PC-HC per se either, but they do negatively affect the WT allele function. Fifteen unique HI variants have been described.[8–10,12,14–18] Only 2 missense variants affecting the same amino acid (N159) have been described to act in a DN manner in humans.[10,11,13,19] HI and DN variants result in distinct clinical and immunologic phenotypes, which are reviewed in this article.

HAPLOINSUFFICIENCY ALLELIC VARIANTS IN IKAROS FAMILY ZINC FINGER 1
Clinical Presentation

Germline heterozygous allelic variants in *IKZF1* acting through a DNA binding to PC-HC HI mechanism have been reported in 59 individuals (30 male) from 19 families[8–10,12,14–18] (see **Fig. 1A**). Clinical manifestations have been described in 43 patients (22 male) with a median age of onset of 11 years (ranging from <1 to 57 years of age) (**Fig. 1B**). Almost one-fourth of *IKZF1* HI mutants were identified in asymptomatic carriers (27.1%, 16 out of 59), suggesting incomplete penetrance of the disease. However, given the wide range of age of initial presentation observed in symptomatic cases, later onset of symptoms cannot be ruled out.

Among the symptomatic patients, bacterial infections were the most frequent clinical manifestation, reported in 79.1% (34 out of 43) of the cases (**Fig. 1C**). The respiratory tract was the system mainly affected, with both upper and lower respiratory tract involvement. Otitis was reported in 23.3% of cases. *Streptococcus pneumoniae* was the most commonly identified pathogen. Patients experienced recurrent episodes of sinopulmonary infections with variable severity. Bronchiectasis has not been described, but chest computed tomography data were scarce in the reports.[8–10,12,14–18]

Sepsis (*S pneumoniae*, *Haemophilus influenzae*, and *Enterococcus gallinarum*) was reported in 5 patients (2 of whom following splenectomy). Four patients, including the 2 splenectomized, had a history of bacterial meningitis caused by *S pneumoniae* and *E gallinarum* infections. Less commonly affected sites for bacterial infections were the skin (3 patients) and the hip joint (1 patient). Chronic or recurrent diarrhea have been described in 4 patients (*Clostridium difficile* and *Blastocystis hominis* identified in 1 patient and *Giardia lamblia* in another). Mycobacterial infection has been reported only in 1 patient, who presented with skin nodules positive for *Mycobacterium chelonae* after receiving chemotherapy for leukemia treatment. Because of myelosuppression, this patient required a bone marrow transplant to control his infection.[9]

Viral infections were described in 4 patients (9.3% of symptomatic cases), generally not severe (herpes simplex virus causing recurrent herpes labialis in 3, human papillomavirus causing warts in hands/feet in 2, and mumps meningitis in 1).[9,10,18] Fungal infections have not been described in *IKZF1* HI (see **Fig. 1**C). Autoimmunity/immune dysregulation was the second most common clinical manifestation described, affecting 39.5% (17 out of 43) of the symptomatic cases. Gender bias was not observed among patients presenting with autoimmunity. Autoimmune conditions started predominantly in childhood, with a median age of clinical presentation of 11 years. Idiopathic thrombocytopenic purpura (ITP) was the most frequently reported (6 patients), followed by systemic lupus erythematosus (SLE in 3 patients).[9,10,12,15–18] Other autoimmune manifestations reported are described in **Table 1**.

Two patients developed B-ALL, at 3 and 5 years of age.[9] A third patient was diagnosed with a solid pseudopapillary pancreas tumor at the age of 22 years.[14]

A distinct presentation of premature birth and nonautoimmune congenital pancytopenia has been documented in 2 unrelated patients sharing the same *IKZF1* variant (p.Y210C).[8,10] To this date, this variant is the sole reported in ZF4 of *IKZF1*. The variant was also detected in an asymptomatic brother of 1 of the probands. This genotype-phenotype correlation suggests unique functions of ZF4 in hematopoiesis, but further studies are needed to better understand the connection.

Laboratory Phenotype

Decreased serum immunoglobulin (Ig) G levels and reduced B-cell counts in peripheral blood were the predominant findings, present in 87.8% (36 out of 41)

Table 1
Autoimmune/ immune dysregulation manifestations in IKAROS haploinsufficiency

Manifestation	Frequency (% of Total Mutation Carriers)
Immune thrombocytopenia	6 (10)
Arthritis	4 (7)
Reactive arthritis (2)	—
Juvenile idiopathic arthritis (1)	—
Seronegative arthritis (1)	—
SLE	3 (5)
Antiphospholipid syndrome	3 (5)
Myasthenia gravis	1 (2)
IgA vasculitis	1 (2)
Urticaria	1 (2)
Hashimoto thyroiditis	1 (2)
Psoriasis-like disease	1 (2)

and 82.9% (34 out of 41) of the symptomatic patients. Among asymptomatic mutation carriers whose laboratorial information was available, 63.6% (7 out of 11) showed a reduction in serum IgG levels, and 42% (5 out of 12) had low B-cell counts, suggesting that immunologic penetrance was observed without clinical manifestations. Longitudinal data from patients who started follow-up at an early age documented a progressive decline in peripheral B-cell counts as well as serum IgG levels.[8–10,12,14–18]

Serum levels of other immunoglobulin isotypes were also reduced (low IgM in 75.7%, 28 out of 37; low IgA in 83.3%, 30 out of 36). Antibody responses to protein as well as polysaccharide vaccines were reduced or absent in most patients tested.[8–10,12,14–18]

In contrast to the B-cell compartment, total T-cell numbers were normal or high in 55.6% (20 out of 36) and 38.9% (14 out of 36) of the patients, respectively. Interestingly, there was a trend toward increased CD8+ T cells, resulting in an inverted CD4/CD8 ratio in 63.4% (26 out of 41) of the patients. This finding was statistically more frequent among patients with protein positive missense mutations than among individual with *IKZF1* full gene deletion.[8] Memory T-cell differentiation, including regulatory T (Treg) and T-follicular helper cells, and proliferation studies, when performed, were mostly normal; however, high and low values have also been reported.[8–10,12,14–18] Natural killer cell numbers were reduced in 30% (6 out of 20) of patients.

Bone marrow studies from a subset of patients with *IKZF1* HI revealed a profound decrease in B-cell lineage precursors or hematogones. Frequencies of hematopoietic stem cells and common lymphoid progenitors were variable. The maturation profile within the B-cell lineage also varied, with some patients showing normal development and others showing a partial to almost complete block at different stages. A very early arrest on B-cell development defined by a marked decrease in pro-B cells (based on the coexpression of cluster of differentiation [CD] 34 and CD19) and even earlier precursors (pre–pro-B cells expressing surface CD34 and cytoplasmic terminal deoxynucleotidyl transferase in the absence of CD19), was characteristically seen in some of these patients.[9,10,12] Moreover, Kuehn and colleagues[9] found normal numbers of CD138+ plasma cells in the bone marrow aspirates from 2 patients with *IKZF1* HI. The investigators hypothesized that the presence of plasma cells in the context of a B-cell maturation arrest may reflect the progressive nature of the disease and may also explain the remnant production of functional antibodies earlier in life.

Treatments and Outcomes

Most patients were treated with broad-spectrum antimicrobial therapy only during acute infectious episodes, although antibiotic prophylaxis was also used. Immunoglobulin replacement, either intravenously or subcutaneously, was the main prophylactic intervention, administered to 56% (19 out of 34) of patients with a history of recurrent or severe bacterial infections. Consistent with a predominantly humoral deficiency, most patients experienced a reduction in frequency and severity of infections after initiation of immunoglobulin substitution.[8–10,12,14–18]

Immune thrombocytopenia was managed with multiple therapeutic approaches, including corticosteroids, high-dose intravenous immunoglobulin, anti-IgD therapy, and rituximab. One patient required splenectomy. Patients with antiphospholipid syndrome received anticoagulation and steroids. Immunosuppressant therapies for SLE included methylprednisolone pulse, hydroxychloroquine, and mycophenolate mofetil.[9,10,12,15–18]

Hematopoietic stem cell transplant (HSCT) was indicated for the 2 patients with nonautoimmune congenital pancytopenia but only performed in 1. The transplanted patient passed away on day 40 post-HSCT because of multiorgan failure, whereas the second patient experienced a spontaneous hematologic recovery after 1 month of birth and did not require HSCT. Despite the overall improvement, his low B-cell level and hypogammaglobulinemia persisted.[8,10]

Out of the 59 *IKZF1* HI mutation carriers reported, 3 are deceased (2 pediatric and 1 adult patient).[8,9] In addition to the previously mentioned infant with pancytopenia who died shortly after HSCT, the second pediatric patient died at 5 years of age of relapsed ALL. The third patient died of pneumonia at the age of 74 years.

DOMINANT NEGATIVE ALLELIC VARIANTS IN IKAROS FAMILY ZINC FINGER 1
Clinical Presentation

Germline dominant allelic variants in *IKZF1* acting through a DN mechanism have been reported in 8 unrelated patients (1 male). No asymptomatic cases have been described. Initial clinical symptoms presented early in life in all patients, ranging from 2 months to 1.5 years of age[10,11,13,19] (see **Fig. 1B**).

The clinical phenotype was characterized by recurrent and severe infections, caused by a broad range of pathogens.[10,11,13,19] All patients presented at least 1 episode of *Pneumocystis jirovecii* pneumonia (PJP) within the first 2 years of life. Two patients experienced multiple episodes of PJP. Recurrent bacterial sinopulmonary infections were reported in 6 out of 8 patients (see **Fig. 1C**). One patient had a history of *S pneumoniae* meningitis. Three patients reported recurrent otitis media and 1 patient skin abscesses. Two cases of mycobacterial infections have been described. One patient had pulmonary *Mycobacterium avium* complex and a second patient developed *Mycobacterium avium intracellulare* lymphadenitis after HSCT. Recurrent or severe viral infections were reported in two-thirds of patients (6 out of 8), including respiratory syncytial virus, adenovirus, influenza, herpes simplex virus, and molluscum contagiosum. Three patients reported chickenpox without complications. In addition to PJP, both superficial (recurrent oral candidiasis) and invasive (pulmonary aspergillosis, *Candida parapsilosis* fungemia) fungal infections have been described. One patient had *Cryptosporidium* species cholangitis that led to cirrhosis.

One patient developed T-cell ALL at the age of 13 years.[11] Autoimmunity, immune dysregulation, or allergic manifestations have not been observed among the reported cases (**Fig. 2**).

Laboratory Phenotype

All patients presented with profound hypogammaglobulinemia involving all major isotypes and nearly absence of peripheral blood B cells.[10,11,13,19] Bone marrow studies performed in 2 DN patients found, similarly to what was described for the patients with HI,[8] an early B-cell developmental arrest with absence of early B-cell precursors. However, in opposition to the patients with HI, plasma cells were virtually absent, suggesting an earlier in life and more severe B-cell maturation arrest in patients carrying *IKZF1* DN mutations.[13]

T-cell counts were variable among patients. Phenotypically, a large predominance of naive T cells presenting features of recent thymic emigrants (ie, CD31+) and T-helper 0 (Th0) phenotype (intracellular interleukin [IL]-2 was detected, but IL-4, interferon gamma, FoxP3, and IL-17 were almost absent), along with a reduction in memory/effector T cells was characteristically observed in all but 1 patient. Moreover, in vitro, patients' T cells failed to acquire a memory phenotype despite appropriate

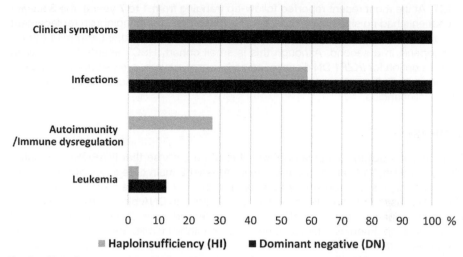

Fig. 2. Clinical presentation of IKAROS-associated primary immunodeficiency by mechanism of action. Percentage indicates penetrance of clinical disease in IKAROS mutation carriers.

stimulation. T-cell receptor (TCR)–driven proliferation was normal in response to strong stimuli, but markedly impaired on low-dose stimulation, and this defect could not be rescued by addition of IL-2. Natural killer cell counts were normal in most patients (71%).[10,11,13,19]

In addition to adaptive immunity defects, disease progression was shown to include myeloid abnormalities, such as eosinopenia and neutropenia, that were distinctively detected in most patients. In vitro studies also showed monocyte dysfunction.[13] Interestingly, the lack of B cells, antibodies, IgE, memory/effector T cells, and eosinophils may play a protective role toward developing allergic and autoimmune/immune dysregulated manifestations in these patients.

Treatments and Outcomes

Because of the earlier and more severe nature of infections seen in this group of patients, all were treated with aggressive antimicrobial regimens and immunoglobulin replacement since very early in life.[10,11,13,19] One patient developed bronchiectasis despite maintenance of appropriate IgG trough levels.[10] Furthermore, because of the life-threatening characteristic of this allelic variant, several patients underwent HSCT based on their clinical/immunophenotypic presentation, as their genetic diagnosis was only retrospectively confirmed.

Kellner and colleagues[19] reported the detailed HSCT outcomes in 4 patients with DN *IKZF1* mutations. One of the patients reported in this series had previously rejected an unconditioned haploidentical CD34+ HSCT at 10 months of age recommended because of combined immunodeficiency. She underwent a second transplant after being diagnosed with T-cell ALL at the age of 13 years. All 4 patients achieved greater than 99% donor chimerism. Infectious complications after transplant included Epstein-Barr virus reactivation in 1, cytomegalovirus viremia in 2, and mycobacterial lymphadenitis in 1 patient. Grade II, skin stage 3, and gastrointestinal tract stage 1 acute graft-versus-host disease (GVHD) was observed in only 1 patient, who responded well to standard treatment. One patient with prior history of *Cryptosporidium* cholangitis progressed to liver failure and died approximately 1 year after

HSCT. At the most recent reported follow-up (ranging from 1 to 7 years), the 3 surviving patients had no signs of chronic GVHD and were off immunoglobulin replacement and antimicrobial prophylaxis. Neutropenia was noticed in 1 patient and mild thrombocytopenia in a second. Although this is small cohort, HSCT seems to be a valid curative option for *IKZF1* DN disease, an early-onset, severe, progressive immunodeficiency with T, B, and myeloid involvement, and increased susceptibility to hematologic malignancies.

SUMMARY

As a crucial regulator of hematopoiesis, it is of no surprise that IKAROS-associated diseases go beyond cancer predisposition. At least 2 main categories of primary immunodeficiencies are caused by autosomal dominant germline mutations in *IKZF1*. Heterozygous *IKZF1* variants acting by HI and affecting DNA binding to PC-HC result in a predominantly antibody deficiency characterized by a CVID-like phenotype of recurrent sinopulmonary infections, hypogammaglobulinemia, and defective vaccine responses with low peripheral B-cell counts and increased risk of autoimmunity and cancer. In contrast, defects dependent on heterozygous DN mutations affecting DNA binding to PC-HC result in an early-onset combined immunodeficiency with recurrent and severe bacterial, viral, and fungal infections and a particular susceptibility to pneumocystis pneumonia. In the latter scenario, the findings of profoundly low B-cell count and predominance of naive T cells serve as diagnostic cues.

The differences in immunologic involvement and clinical phenotypes between HI and DN allelic variants affecting DNA binding to PC-HC suggest an *IKZF1* gene dosage and type of mutation effect. Patients with HI mutations caused by a single-gene full deletion seemed to have a less extended immunologic lineage impact than those with single-gene missense mutations. Although patients with single-gene full deletions make up ~50% of WT/WT IKZF1 homodimers (all produced by their remaining WT allele) and show an almost exclusive B-cell impact, patients carrying single-gene missense mutations form ~25% of WT/WT homodimers (the rest being ~50% WT/mutant, and ~25% mutant/mutant) and present with a B-cell plus a CD8+ T-cell and dendritic cell involvement.[9,21] Moreover, patients carrying the more aggressive DN mutations show a deleterious effect not only on B-cell development but also on T cells (arrested at a naive/Th0 stage with virtually no Th1/Th2/Th17/Treg commitment, and defective TCR signaling), and myeloid cells (neutropenia, eosinopenia, and monocyte dysfunction).[13] In other words, and based on the clinical immune phenotypes of patients with HI and DN status, B cells seem to be the most sensitive and myeloid cells (in general) the least sensitive lineages to *IKZF1* gene dosage.[9,13,21,22]

So far, both somatic as well as germline *IKZF1* genetic defects have been described to be associated with different clinical phenotypes affecting the hematopoietic compartment. A combination of malignant lymphoproliferative diseases (eg, leukemias), central cytopenias (eg, B-cell lymphopenia), autoimmunity/immune dysregulation (eg, ITP and SLE), and immunodeficiency manifestations characterized by increased infectious disease susceptibility, all with variable degrees of expressivity, have been associated with those mutations. However, although this article addresses the pathophysiology, clinical manifestations, and laboratory manifestations, as well as penetrance and expressivity of genetic variants affecting IKAROS' N-terminal ZFs directly involved in DNA binding to PC-HC, it is likely that this description only represents a partial view of the evolving picture of IKAROS-associated diseases. Defects affecting the C-terminal ZFs directly involved in protein dimerization have not been described to date, and neither have mutations behaving as gain of function or displaying neomorphic activities. Although this hypothesis could sound far-fetched, a scenario depicting multiple allelic variants and immune phenotypes associated with a single gene has been already described for other transcription factors, as in signal transducer and activator of transcription (STAT) 1 and STAT3.[23–25] Unless these yet-to-be described *IKZF1* changes are intrinsically incompatible with life (not suggested by the animal models representing some of these defects), it is possible that such experiments of nature[26] will be diagnosed in the future. In order for that to happen, unbiased genetic diagnostic approaches to evaluate patients with PID/inborn errors of immunity must be pursued, in opposition to a clinical manifestations-based candidate gene diagnosis strategy, which has already proved us wrong multiple times. Furthermore, testing all symptomatic and asymptomatic relatives to the index patients in a systematic way should be pursued as the proper way of determining the spectrum, penetrance, and expressivity of these diseases.

ACKNOWLEDGMENTS

This work was supported by the Intramural Research Program, National Institutes of Health Clinical Center. The content of this article does not necessarily reflect the views or policies of the Department of Health and Human Services, nor does mention of trade names, commercial products, or organizations imply endorsement by the US government.

DISCLOSURE OF POTENTIAL CONFLICT OF INTEREST

The authors have no relevant conflicts of interest.

REFERENCES

1. Georgopoulos K, Moore DD, Derfler B. Ikaros, an early lymphoid-specific transcription factor and a putative mediator for T cell commitment. Science 1992; 258(5083):808–12.
2. Georgopoulos K, Bigby M, Wang JH, et al. The Ikaros gene is required for the development of all lymphoid lineages. Cell 1994;79(1):143–56.
3. Yoshida T, Georgopoulos K. Ikaros fingers on lymphocyte differentiation. Int J Hematol 2014;100(3):220–9.
4. Francis OL, Payne JL, Su RJ, et al. Regulator of myeloid differentiation and function: The secret life of Ikaros. World J Biol Chem 2011;2(6):119–25.
5. Kastner P, Dupuis A, Gaub MP, et al. Function of Ikaros as a tumor suppressor in B cell acute lymphoblastic leukemia. Am J Blood Res 2013;3(1):1–13.
6. Mullighan CG, Su X, Zhang J, et al. Deletion of IKZF1 and prognosis in acute lymphoblastic leukemia. N Engl J Med 2009;360(5):470–80.
7. Churchman ML, Qian M, Te Kronnie G, et al. Germline Genetic IKZF1 Variation and Predisposition to Childhood Acute Lymphoblastic Leukemia. Cancer Cell 2018;33(5):937–48.e8.
8. Goldman FD, Gurel Z, Al-Zubeidi D, et al. Congenital pancytopenia and absence of B lymphocytes in a neonate with a mutation in the Ikaros gene. Pediatr Blood Cancer 2012;58(4):591–7.
9. Kuehn HS, Boisson B, Cunningham-Rundles C, et al. Loss of B cells in patients with heterozygous mutations in IKAROS. N Engl J Med 2016;374(11):1032–43.

10. Hoshino A, Okada S, Yoshida K, et al. Abnormal hematopoiesis and autoimmunity in human subjects with germline IKZF1 mutations. J Allergy Clin Immunol 2017; 140(1):223–31.
11. Yoshida N, Sakaguchi H, Muramatsu H, et al. Germline IKAROS mutation associated with primary immunodeficiency that progressed to T-cell acute lymphoblastic leukemia. Leukemia 2017;31(5):1221–3.
12. Bogaert DJ, Kuehn HS, Bonroy C, et al. A novel IKAROS haploinsufficiency kindred with unexpectedly late and variable B-cell maturation defects. J Allergy Clin Immunol 2018;141(1):432–5.e7.
13. Boutboul D, Kuehn HS, Van de Wyngaert Z, et al. Dominant-negative IKZF1 mutations cause a T, B, and myeloid cell combined immunodeficiency. J Clin Invest 2018;128(7):3071–87.
14. Chen QY, Wang XC, Wang WJ, et al. B-cell deficiency: a De Novo IKZF1 patient and review of the literature. J Investig Allergol Clin Immunol 2018;28(1):53–6.
15. Sriaroon P, Chang Y, Ujhazi B, et al. Familial immune thrombocytopenia associated with a novel variant in IKZF1. Front Pediatr 2019;7:139.
16. Van Nieuwenhove E, Garcia-Perez JE, Helsen C, et al. A kindred with mutant IKAROS and autoimmunity. J Allergy Clin Immunol 2018;142(2):699–702.e2.
17. Eskandarian Z, Fliegauf M, Bulashevska A, et al. Assessing the functional relevance of variants in the IKAROS family zinc finger protein 1 (IKZF1) in a cohort of patients with primary immunodeficiency. Front Immunol 2019;10:568.
18. Dieudonné Y, Guffroy A, Vollmer O, et al. IKZF1 loss-of-function variant causes autoimmunity and severe familial antiphospholipid syndrome. J Clin Immunol 2019;39(4):353–7.
19. Kellner ES, Krupski C, Kuehn HS, et al. Allogeneic hematopoietic stem cell transplant outcomes for patients with dominant negative IKZF1/IKAROS mutations. J Allergy Clin Immunol 2019;144(1):339–42.
20. John LB, Ward AC. The Ikaros gene family: transcriptional regulators of hematopoiesis and immunity. Mol Immunol 2011;48(9–10):1272–8.
21. Cytlak U, Resteu A, Bogaert D, et al. Ikaros family zinc finger 1 regulates dendritic cell development and function in humans. Nat Commun 2018;9(1):1239.
22. Abdulhay N, Fiorini C, Kumánovics A, et al. Normal hematologic parameters and fetal hemoglobin silencing with heterozygous IKZF1 mutations. Blood 2016; 128(16):2100–3.
23. Olbrich P, Freeman AF. STAT1 and STAT3 mutations: important lessons for clinical immunologists. Expert Rev Clin Immunol 2018;14(12):1029–41.
24. Jhamnani RD, Rosenzweig SD. An update on gain-of-function mutations in primary immunodeficiency diseases. Curr Opin Allergy Clin Immunol 2017;17(6): 391–7.
25. Shahmarvand N, Nagy A, Shahryari J, et al. Mutations in the signal transducer and activator of transcription family of genes in cancer. Cancer Sci 2018; 109(4):926–33.
26. Good RA, Zak SJ. Disturbances in gamma globulin synthesis as experiments of nature. Pediatrics 1956;18(1):109–49.

Asplenia and Hyposplenism
An Underrecognized Immune Deficiency

Jacqueline D. Squire, MD, Mandel Sher, MD*

KEYWORDS

- Asplenia • Hyposplenism • Immune deficiency
- Overwhelming postsplenectomy infection • Invasive pneumococcal disease

KEY POINTS

- Asplenia and hyposplenism may occur in a multitude of different disorders but often is not assessed during immune evaluation.
- In conditions associated with asplenia or hyposplenism, an evaluation of splenic function should be obtained starting with peripheral smear for Howell-Jolly bodies. For patients with high suspicion of splenic dysfunction, further evaluation with pitted red blood cell count or technetium Tc 99m–labeled scintigraphy should be considered.
- Asplenia and hyposplenism increase the risk of infection, especially invasive pneumococcal disease.
- Approaches to prevent infection in asplenic patients include patient education, vaccination, and antibiotic prophylaxis.

INTRODUCTION

Asplenia and hyposplenism often are thought of as rare conditions, and evaluation of splenic function seldom is obtained during evaluation for immune deficiency. Over the past several decades, with improvement in measures of splenic function, the number of known disorders associated with asplenia and functional hyposplenism has grown (**Table 1**). The importance of identifying splenic dysfunction is to recognize those at increased risk of infection, especially invasive pneumococcal disease (IPD). A recent study by Scheuerman and colleagues[1] evaluated 74 children with various complaints, predominantly persistent thrombocytosis and recurrent/severe infections, and found that more than half of the patients had evidence of impaired splenic function. The rates of IPD have decreased significantly since introduction of pneumococcal vaccination, to the point that presentation of severe IPD in a fully vaccinated child should prompt consideration for evaluation of immune deficiency.[2]

Division of Allergy and Immunology, Department of Pediatrics, Morsani College of Medicine, University of South Florida, 601 4th Street South, CRI 4008, St Petersburg, FL 33701, USA
* Corresponding author.
E-mail address: Jacquelinesquire7@gmail.com

Immunol Allergy Clin N Am 40 (2020) 471–483
https://doi.org/10.1016/j.iac.2020.03.006
immunology.theclinics.com

Table 1
Causes of asplenia and functional hyposplenia

Congenital	Rheumatologic
Isolated congenital asplenia	SLE
Heterotaxy syndrome	Hashimoto thyroiditis
APECED	Graves disease
Stormorken syndrome	Multiple sclerosis
Hematologic/oncologic	Rheumatoid arthritis
Sickle hemoglobinopathies	Sarcoidosis
Hereditary spherocytosis	Wegener granulomatosis
Leukemia	Goodpasture syndrome
Lymphoma	Sjögren syndrome
Systemic mastocytosis	Glomerulonephritis
Chronic myeloproliferative disorders	Immunologic
Fanconi syndrome	Severe combined immune deficiency
Hematopoietic cell transplant	C2 deficiency
Graft-versus-host disease	IRAK-4 deficiency
Gastrointestinal	IgG2-IgG4 deficiency
Celiac disease	IgA deficiency
Inflammatory bowel disease	Infectious disease
Autoimmune atropic gastritis	Human Immunodeficiency virus/AIDS
Autoimmune enteropathy	Miscellaneous
Eosinophilic gastrointestinal disorders	Amyloidosis
Whipple disease	Circulatory
Intestinal lymphangiectasia	Splenic artery thrombosis
Hepatic	Splenic vein thrombosis
Autoimmune hepatitis	Celiac artery thrombosis
Liver cirrhosis	Iatrogenic
Alcoholic liver disease	High-dose corticosteroids
Primary biliary cirrhosis	Methyldopa
Primary sclerosing cholangitis	Total parental nutrition
	Splenic irradiation

Adapted from William BM, Corazza GR. Hyposplenism: a comprehensive review. Part I: basic concepts and causes. Hematology 2007;12(1):1-13; and Di Sabatino A, Carsetti R, Corazza GR. Post-splenectomy and hyposplenic states. Lancet 2011;378(9785):90.

CAUSES OF ASPLENIA AND HYPOSPLENISM

Assessment of splenic function should be considered in these cases as well, given that the rate of asplenia in children with recurrent invasive pneumococcal infections has been reported as up to 8.3%.[3]

This review highlights the anatomy and function of the spleen, methods of assessing splenic function, disorders associated with asplenia and hyposplenism, complications of splenic dysfunction, and recommendations for prevention of infection in this population.

FUNCTION AND ANATOMY OF THE SPLEEN

The spleen is the largest lymphoid organ of the body. Its major function is to filter the blood, removing pathogens and undesired particles, such as erythrocyte inclusion bodies and immune complexes.[4,5] The spleen is composed of distinct anatomic regions, known as the red pulp, the white pulp, and the marginal zone. The red pulp contains primarily vascular sinusoids and is the principal area of filtration whereby red pulp macrophages remove microbes and damaged or worn-out cells.[5] The red pulp macrophages can directly recognize some bacteria but rely mainly on opsonization by complement or opsonizing molecules, such as properdin or tuftsin, which are produced by the spleen.[6] The white pulp is composed of lymphocytes, segregated into T-cell and B-cell zones, similar to lymph nodes. The boundary between the red pulp and the white pulp is referred to as the marginal zone.[5] B cells in the marginal zone express high levels of IgM and complement receptor 2, enabling rapid T-independent B-cell activation and immunoglobulin secretion.[7] The spleen is home to a unique population of B cells within the marginal zone, called IgM memory B cells. These cells are thought to help initiate the immune response against encapsulated bacteria, such as *Streptococcus pneumoniae*, *Neisseria meningitidis*, and *Haemophilus influenzae* type b, which are not well opsonized by complement.[6,8]

ASSESSING SPLENIC FUNCTION

Identifying patients with splenic dysfunction, without known history of splenectomy or congenital asplenia, can be difficult due to the lack of easily attainable measures of splenic function. The most well-known form of evaluation is identification of Howell-Jolly bodies within erythrocytes on peripheral blood smear. These inclusion bodies are DNA particles that remain after the nucleus is expelled from erythrocyte precursor cells. The spleen typically removes these nuclear particles, or the entire erythrocyte, as blood is filtered through the vascular sinusoids.[9] Greater than 1% Howell-Jolly body–containing erythrocytes on peripheral smear indicates splenic dysfunction.[10] This method often is not considered reliable, however, due to user error or small number of cells counted and because the absence of Howell-Jolly bodies does not indicate normal splenic function.[1,10–13] Measurement by flow cytometry has been developed on a research basis.[10,14]

Additional hematologic abnormalities can be visualized on peripheral smear in patients with splenic dysfunction, including acanthocytes, target cells, Heinz bodies, siderocytes, or iron granules.[1,9] Leukocytosis and thrombocytosis also are common findings on complete blood cell count.[1,15] The most sensitive hematologic indicator of splenic function, however, is counting pitted erythrocytes (**Fig. 1**). These pits are vacuoles in the plasma membrane of erythrocytes that accumulate with age.[9,16] This method has been shown to correlate with varying degrees of hyposplenism.

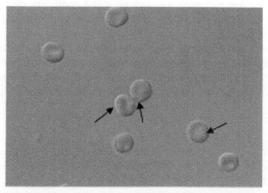

Fig. 1. Pitted erythrocyte images. Pits within cell membrane of erythrocytes (*arrows*) viewed with differential interference contrast. (*Courtesy of* Jennifer Korpik, MT (ASCP) with the CBDI Erythrocyte Diagnostic Laboratory at Cincinnati Children's Hospital Medical Center, Cincinnati, OH.)

Erythrocyte pit counts of 0% to 4% are considered normal, with values above 4% indicating splenic dysfunction and values of greater than 15% to 16% consistent with asplenia or clinically significant hyposplenism.[13,16,17] Pitted erythrocyte counts also have been shown to correlate with scintigraphic measurements of splenic function and have a sensitivity, specificity, and predictive value all between 90% to 98%.[13,17–19] The downside to this method is that it requires specialized electron microscopy.[11] This test, red blood cell pit count, is commercially available through Cincinnati Children's Erythrocyte Diagnostic Laboratory.

Another accepted method for examination of splenic function is technetium Tc 99m (^{99m}Tc)-labeled sulfur colloid, or autologous erythrocyte, liver-spleen scintigraphy.[9,16] This method assesses the spleen's ability to filter by measuring the clearance rate of radiolabeled colloid or erythrocytes. Scintigraphy also can be combined with single-photon emission computed tomography and low-dose computed tomography to calculate the splenic functional volume.[13] Autologous erythrocytes now often are preferred over sulfur colloid due to the lower rate of liver uptake with erythrocyte scintigraphy.[9,13] The disadvantage of this method is it is more invasive, expensive, and exposes the patient to radiation.

Immunologic assessment of splenic function has been described. The spleen is a primary source for production of certain opsonin peptides, such as tuftsin, which can be measured in the serum. Decreased levels have been found in patients after splenectomy, in those with sickle cell disease, and in celiac disease.[9] Another unique marker of immunologic function of the spleen is IgM memory B cells. These non–class-switched memory B cells require the spleen for generation and survival. Splenectomized and asplenic patients have significantly reduced IgM memory B-cell levels compared with normal, and this reduction is associated with increased pneumococcal infection frequency.[8]

A stepwise approach to evaluation of splenic function may be the most cost-effective and judicious method. A peripheral smear for evaluation of Howell-Jolly bodies should be considered in all patients with a risk of asplenia or functional hyposplenism (see **Table 1**). If present, the patient can be considered functionally asplenic/hyposplenic and appropriate preventative measures initiated. If Howell-Jolly bodies are not present, this does not rule out splenic dysfunction, and further evaluation should be considered in high-risk patients. The next appropriate method to obtain, if or when available, is pitted erythrocyte count. In patients with high suspicion and inability to obtain, or inconclusive, results with the methods discussed previously, ^{99m}Tc-labeled autologous erythrocyte scintigraphy, is considered the definitive measurement of splenic function.[9]

Functional asplenia and hyposplenism have been described in a wide variety of disorders, associated with almost every organ system (see **Table 1**). Although the most common cause of asplenia is surgical removal of the spleen,[15] some of the most well-known disorders associated with asplenia and functional hyposplenism are highlighted.

Congenital

Isolated congenital asplenia, without additional anatomic defects, is a rare disorder that has been described mainly in case reports in the literature. One large nationwide French study estimated the prevalence to be 0.51 per million births.[20] Isolated congenital asplenia has been referred to as a primary immune deficiency because it leaves patients particularly susceptible to overwhelming pneumococcal infection throughout life.[20,21] Recently, mutations in RPSA have been implicated as a cause for congenital asplenia in humans.[22,23]

Another congenital cause of asplenia is heterotaxy syndrome, referring to a group of disorders with abnormal thoracoabdominal organ arrangement due to right or left isomerism, commonly associated with congenital heart defects.[24] Previously, heterotaxy associated with splenic abnormalities (agenesis, malposition, and multiple spleens) was known as Ivemark syndrome, after the physician who initial described this disorder in 1955.[15,25] Heterotaxy syndrome is used interchangeably with asplenia or polysplenia syndrome. Traditionally, asplenia is associated with right isomerism whereas polysplenia is associated with left isomerism though these terms often are used interchangeably with the rotational defect regardless of assessment of splenic status.[24,26] Despite having multiple spleens, patients with polysplenia may have functional hyposplenism and appear to be at increased risk of infection with encapsulated bacteria similar to patients with asplenia.[27] Heterotaxy syndrome is much more common than congenital asplenia, diagnosed in approximately 1 in 5000 to 7000 live births, although not all defects involve in the spleen.[24] Mutations in connexin 43 and ZIC3 are associated with heterotaxy syndromes.[21]

Asplenia is described in other genetic disorders, including autoimmune polyendocrinopathy-candidiasis-ectodermal dystrophy (APECED), also known as autoimmune polyglandular syndrome type 1. APECED is an autosomal recessive disorder due to defects in the AIRE gene, resulting in a variable presentation of autoimmunity, endocrinopathy, ectodermal dystrophy, and susceptlbility to infection with Candida.[15] Patients with APECED have been reported to have complete asplenia or functional hyposplenism, as determined by lack of radiolabeled colloid uptake on technetium scan. Functional hyposplenism appears to worsen with age in some patients, indicating loss of splenic function may be autoimmune.[28,29] Another genetic cause of asplenia is Storkmorken syndrome due to defects in STIM1. In addition to asplenia, patients present with tubular aggregate myopathy, thrombocytopenia or platelet dysfunction, miosis, ichthyosis, short stature, dyslexia, and migraines.[30]

Hematologic/Oncologic

The most well-studied acquired cause of functional asplenia is sickle cell anemia. With the decline in fetal hemoglobin after birth, sickled cells begin accumulating in the slow circulatory system of the spleen causing initial enlargement of the organ. Over time, recurrent sickling of cells within the spleen leads to splenic infarction and autosplenectomy by midchildhood.[15] Evidence of splenic dysfunction starts as early as 6 months of age and by 5 years more than 90% of children with sickle cell anemia have functional hyposplenism. The increased risk of IPD in young children with sickle anemia is attributed to the combination of early loss of splenic function and a naïve immune system.[15,19]

Decreased splenic function has been reported in a variety of malignancies, due either to direct tumor infiltration of the spleen or to consequences of treatment.[15] Functional hyposplenism has been described in 15% to 40% of patients after bone marrow transplant.[6] Chronic graft-versus-host disease post-transplant also increases the risk hyposplenism and pneumococcal sepsis.[15,31]

Gastrointestinal

A recognized association between celiac disease and splenic dysfunction exists. Hyposplenism is prevalent in 16% to 76% of adults with celiac disease, depending on the method used to assess splenic function.[6,15] The development of hyposplenism has been associated with the duration of exposure to dietary gluten and as such is less common in children with celiac disease.[15,32] Patients with autoimmune disorder–associated celiac disease also are reported to have significantly increased risk of hyposplenism compared with those without autoimmune features.[33] The clinical importance of hyposplenism in this disorder was confirmed in a recent systemic review and meta-analysis by Simons and colleagues,[34] demonstrating that the odds of pneumococcal infection in celiac disease is approximately double that of controls. Although some patients may be affected by irreversible splenic atrophy, functional hyposplenism has been shown to improve with a gluten-free diet.[6,15,32]

Approximately 40% of patients with inflammatory bowel disease demonstrate evidence of hyposplenism with elevated pitted erythrocyte counts and decreased IgM memory B cells.[35] A nationwide Danish cohort study identified that patients with inflammatory bowel disease were at significantly increased risk of IPD compared with controls, from 1.5-fold and 2-fold increased risks for ulcerative colitis and Crohn's disease, respectively.[36] Medical or surgical treatment of ulcerative colitis can improve splenic function, although similar to celiac disease, splenic atrophy often is irreversible.[15] Recently, 2 studies have identified an increased risk of hyposplenism in other gastrointestinal disorders, including primary eosinophilic disorders (esophagitis, gastroenteritis, or colitis), autoimmune atrophic gastritis, autoimmune enteropathy, and autoimmune liver diseases.[37,38] The rate of pneumococcal infection and clinical implication of hyposplenism for these disorders is not yet known.

Rheumatologic

Hyposplenism and splenic atrophy has been reported in several different autoimmune disorders (see **Table 1**). The reported incidence of hyposplenism from small patient cohorts with systemic lupus erythematous (SLE) ranges widely between 4.6% and 86% with different methods of assessment.[15] SLE-associated hyposplenism also appears to be reversible with treatment in some cases, but irreversible with splenic atrophy.[39] Incidence of hyposplenism in rheumatoid arthritis varies widely between studies, 21% to 85%.[15] A large cohort analysis from England demonstrated that patients with a variety of rheumatologic conditions, including rheumatoid arthritis and SLE, had significantly increased risk of IPD after diagnosis. Patients with SLE had particularly high risk with a rate ratio of 4.4 to 8.9 compared with controls.[40]

Immunologic

Hyposplenism has been described in patients with other forms of immune deficiency. A study by Scheuerman and colleagues[1] demonstrated functional asplenia/hyposplenism in children with severe combined immune deficiency, complement C2 deficiency, interleukin-1 receptor–associated kinase-4 (IRAK-4) deficiency, IgG2-IgG4 deficiency, and transient hypogammaglobulinemia. Two of these patients, one with IRAK-4 and one with C2 deficiency, had invasive pneumococcal disease. There has also been 1 report of asplenia with IgA deficiency.[41]

COMPLICATIONS OF SPLENIC DYSFUNCTION
Infection

The complication of greatest concern in patients with asplenia or functional hyposplenism is IPD or overwhelming postsplenectomy infection (OPSI). OPSI refers to sepsis, meningitis, or pneumonia in patients with asplenia and most often is caused by encapsulated bacteria, such as S pneumoniae (>50% of cases), N meningitidis, and H influenzae type b.[6] OPSI may begin with a mild prodrome; however, rapid deterioration and death often occur within 24 hours to 48 hours. The mortality rate in OPSI is up to 50% to 70% due to shock, hypoglycemia, acidosis, respiratory distress, and disseminated intravascular coagulation, with the highest rates in children less than 2 years.[6,42,43] A review of 78 studies found the incidence rates of OPSI in splenectomized adults and children were 3.2% and 3.3%, respectively, during a median follow-up of 6.9 years. Most infections occurred within 2 years of splenectomy, although up to one-third occurred an average of 5 years after.[44] A recent prospective study by Theilacker and colleagues[45] confirmed delayed onset, a median of almost 6 years, of OPSI postsplenectomy. The estimated lifetime risk of OPSI for asplenic patients is 5%, more than 600 times the general population risk, and cases have been reported 20 years to 50 years after splenectomy.[6,45,46] The overall incidence of OPSI or IPD for functional hyposplenism is not known, but increased risk has been documented in heterotaxy syndrome, gastrointestinal, hematologic, and rheumatologic disorders, as discussed previously.[19,27,31,34,36,40,47]

Additional infections of concern in asplenic patients include the intraerythrocytic parasites *Babesia*, *Plasmodium falciparum*, and *Erchilia*.[47,48] Severe sepsis after dog bite due to *Capnocytophaga canimorsus* also has been reported.[48]

Vascular

Venous and arterial vascular complications have been reported in patients postsplenectomy.

The condition for which the splenectomy was performed appears to the have greatest influence on the risk of developing these complications. Certain populations of patients, in particular those with hemoglobinopathies, are reported to have an increased rate of ischemic heart disease and stroke postsplenectomy.[49] Portal vein thrombosis incidence after splenectomy has ranged between 0.7% and 37%. A majority of cases occur shortly after splenic removal, indicating that anatomic or surgical factors may be responsible (the splenic vein drains to the portal vein).[47,49] Additional venous complications reported after splenectomy include deep vein thrombosis and pulmonary embolism. An increased risk of pulmonary arterial hypertension has been documented after splenectomy as well as associated with a case of congenital asplenia.[49,50]

PREVENTION OF INFECTION

The primary objective in treatment of patients with asplenia and functional hyposplenism is preventing infection. Strategies to address the concern of OPSI or IPD include patient education regarding risks and symptoms of infection, vaccination, and antibiotic prophylaxis. Additionally, methods for preserving splenic tissue and function are reviewed.

Education

Patient knowledge of preventative recommendations and complications associated with asplenia and hyposplenism can decrease infectious complications.[51] Patients should receive proper counseling on recommended vaccinations, prophylactic antibiotics, and fever management. To raise awareness, patient registries have been developed to disseminate pertinent information to patients and clinicians. This strategy has been shown to increase the rate of compliance with recommendations.[52] Enrollment in a registry for asplenia/hyposplenism can also significantly improve patient outcomes. The Spleen Australia registry demonstrated a 69% decrease in the rate of IPD and invasive meningococcal disease for patients after registry enrollment, an absolute risk reduction of 5 to 6 invasive infections per year.[53]

Vaccination

Vaccination is a key strategy to preventing invasive infections regardless of immuno-compromise or competency. Thankfully, effective vaccines against *S pneumoniae*, *N meningitidis*, and *H influenzae* type b exist. The Advisory Committee on Immunization Practices and the Infectious Diseases Society of America provide vaccination recommendations for adults and children with immunocompromising conditions, including anatomic or functional asplenia.[54–59] **Table 2** lists these recommendations.

For patients undergoing elective splenectomy, it is recommended that they receive the indicated vaccines at least 2 weeks prior to surgery. In cases of emergency splenectomy, vaccination should be given at least 2 weeks postoperatively.[59,60]

Antibiotic Prophylaxis

Antibiotic prophylaxis has been studied primarily in patients with sickle cell anemia. Prophylaxis until 5 years of age demonstrated significant decrease in IPD whereas continuing past age 5, when risk of IPD is substantially lower, it did not have a significant reduction in disease. Based on these prior studies, is currently is recommended

Table 2	
Vaccination recommendations for patients with anatomic or functional asplenia	

Pneumococcal	• Patients <6 y old should receive primary PCV13 series
	  ◦ PPSV23 given at ≥2 y old, booster dose ≥5 y after first dose
	• Patients ≥6 y old and adults, who have not received PCV13 previously, should receive 1 dose of PCV13, followed by PPSV23 ≥8 wk after
	  ◦ PPSV23 booster ≥5 y after first dose
	  ◦ PPSV23 at ≥65 y[a]

Meningococcal ACWY	• Patients 2–23 mo old should receive primary series with MenACWY-CRM or Hib-MenCY-TT
	  ◦ Initial booster 3 y after primary series, additional boosters every 5 y[b]
	• Patients ≥2 y old and adults, who have not received prior vaccination, should receive primary series with MenACWY-D
	  ◦ Booster every 5 y; if primary series at <7 y old, then initial booster 3 y after primary

Meningococcal B	• Patients ≥10 y old and adults should receive primary series with MenB-4C or MenB-FHbp

H influenzae type b	• Patients <12 mo old should receive primary series
	• Patients 12–59 mo old
	  ◦ 0–1 dose prior to 12 mo: give 2 doses, 8 wk apart
	  ◦ >2 doses prior to 12 mo: give 1 dose, 8 wk after last
	• Patients ≥60 mo old and adults, unimmunized with *H influenzae* type b: give 1 dose

Influenza	• Should receive yearly inactivated flu vaccine

Abbreviations: Hib-MenCY-TT, Haemophilus b and Meningococcal (Groups C, Y), Tetanus Toxoid Conjugate Vaccine (MenHibrix); MenACWY-CRM, quadrivalent meningiococcal (Groups A, C, W-135, Y) conjugate vaccine (Menveo); MenACWY-D, Meningococcal (Groups A, C, Y and W-135) Polysaccharide Diphtheria Toxoid Conjugate Vaccine (Menactra); MenB-FHbp, meningococcal group B vaccine (Trumenba); MenB-4C, meningococcal group B vaccine (Bexsero); PCV13, pneumococcal 13-valent conjugate vaccine (Prevnar 13); PPSV23, pneumococcal polysaccharide vaccine (Pneumovax 23).
[a] Should not receive more than one PPSV23 after 65 y of age.
[b] Booster with MenACWY-CRM or MenACWY-D only.
Data from Refs.[54–59]

that all children up to 5 years old with asplenia or functional hyposplenism receive daily prophylaxis to prevent IPD.[60,61] It also is recommended that older children and adults receive prophylaxis for at least 1 year after splenectomy or lifelong prophylaxis after an episode of postsplenectomy sepsis.[60] Controversy exists regarding the optimal duration of antibiotic prophylaxis though. Canadian guidelines agree with these recommendations, whereas British and Australian guidelines have advocated for longer prophylaxis after splenectomy, up to 3 years or consideration of lifelong prophylaxis in all patients.[43,62]

The preferred prophylactic regimen is penicillin, 125 mg twice a day, for patients less than 3 years old, and 250 mg twice a day, for patients 3 years and older. Amoxicillin, 20 mg/kg per day, is an accepted alternative.[63] Concern for penicillin allergy should prompt referral to an allergist for thorough evaluation because options for penicillin-allergic patients are limited; erythromycin, 250 mg twice a day, is the generally recommended alternative.[43,63] For travel to endemic areas, patients with asplenia or functional hyposplenism should receive malaria prophylaxis. In cases of a dog bite, patients should receive a course of prophylactic antibiotics due to the risk of C canimorsus sepsis.[43,60] If not on daily oral prophylaxis, a 1-time dose should be given prior to minimally invasive and invasive dental procedures. Prophylaxis is not needed prior to routine cleanings.[43,64]

Fever Management

Patients with asplenia or functional hyposplenism require prompt evaluation for fever. Patients should be advised to present to a medical facility within 2 hours of fever for examination, laboratory testing, and blood cultures. If they are well appearing, laboratory tests are reassuring, and proper follow-up is assured, patients may receive a 1-time dose of intravenous or intramuscular ceftriaxone and be discharged. If unable to reach a medical center for evaluation promptly, it is recommended that patients receive a 1-time dose of amoxicillin (this can be prescribed ahead of time for patient to have on hand).[60]

SPLENIC CONSERVATION

With the concern for OPSI and IPD in asplenic patients, methods to conserve splenic function after trauma or ways to avoid splenectomy in other disorders have been proposed. One approach gaining favor is the use if splenic artery embolization (SAE) in hemodynamically stable patients after trauma. This method has demonstrated conservation of not only splenic volume but also immune function, evidenced by preservation of IgM memory B cells after SAE compared with splenectomy.[65]

Chronic immune thrombocytopenia (ITP) is a disorder in which splenectomy may be utilized for treatment refractory patients. Recent studies have been conducted to evaluate alternatives to splenectomy, including rituximab and thrombopoietin receptor agonists. Both of these medications carry a risk of increased infection and thrombosis, respectively; therefore, age and comorbidities should be taken into account when determining appropriate therapy.[66] Additional immune deficiency may increase the risk of infection postsplenectomy significantly. Wong and colleagues[67] demonstrated that splenectomy in patients with common variable immune deficiency results in increased risk of infection with encapsulated bacteria, particularly if not receiving immunoglobulin replacement.

DISCUSSION

Patients with asplenia or functional hyposplenism are at significantly increased risk of infection with encapsulated bacteria, in particular S pneumoniae. Invasive pneumococcal infection should prompt physicians to evaluate for immune deficiency, including evaluation of splenic function.[2,3] Early assessment of splenic function also should be considered in disorders known to be associated with asplenia and functional hyposplenism (see **Table 1**), given recent evidence of increased risk of pneumococcal infections in these populations.[27,31,34,40] In patients with these disorders, a peripheral smear should be obtained to screen for Howell-Jolly bodies. Although detection of Howell-Jolly bodies on peripheral smear is indicative of asplenia or functional hyposplenism, the lack of these inclusion bodies is not sufficient to establish splenic function. Therefore, further evaluation with erythrocyte pit counts or scintigraphy, as available, should be considered in patients with high suspicion of splenic dysfunction, such as those with a history of recurrent or invasive infection with *S pneumoniae*, *N meningitidis*, and *H influenzae* type b. Once patients are identified, methods to decrease their risk of infection should be implemented, including patient education, vaccination, and antibiotic prophylaxis. When splenectomy is considered for trauma or treatment refractory cytopenias, alternatives, such as SAE and immune-modulating agents, respectively, also should be considered.

DISCLOSURE

The authors have nothing to disclose.

REFERENCES

1. Scheuerman O, Bar-Sever Z, Hoffer V, et al. Functional hyposplenism is an important and underdiagnosed immunodeficiency condition in children. Acta Paediatr 2014;103(9):e399–403.
2. Gaschignard J, Levy C, Chrabieh M, et al. Invasive pneumococcal disease in children can reveal a primary immunodeficiency. Clin Infect Dis 2014;59(2):244–51.
3. Butters C, Phuong LK, Cole T, et al. Prevalence of Immunodeficiency in Children With Invasive Pneumococcal Disease in the Pneumococcal Vaccine Era: A Systematic Review. JAMA Pediatr 2019;173(11):1084–94.
4. Ballow M. Stress-related immunodeficiencies: trauma, surgery, anesthesia, burns, exercise, and splenic deficiencies. In: Stiehm ER, Ochs HD, Winkelstein JA, editors. Immunologic disorders in infants & children. 5th edition. Philadelphia: Elsevier; 2004. p. 956–60.
5. Abbas AK, LA, Pillai S. Cells and tissues of the immune system. In: Abbas AK, Lichtman AHH, Pillai S, editors. Cellular and molecular immunology. 9th edition. Philadelphia: Elsevier; 2018. p. 35–6.
6. Di Sabatino A, Carsetti R, Corazza GR. Post-splenectomy and hyposplenic states. Lancet 2011;378(9785):86–97.
7. Weller S, Braun MC, Tan BK, et al. Human blood IgM "memory" B cells are circulating splenic marginal zone B cells harboring a prediversified immunoglobulin repertoire. Blood 2004;104(12):3647–54.
8. Kruetzmann S, Rosado MM, Weber H, et al. Human immunoglobulin M memory B cells controlling Streptococcus pneumoniae infections are generated in the spleen. J Exp Med 2003;197(7):939–45.
9. de Porto AP, Lammers AJ, Bennink RJ, et al. Assessment of splenic function. Eur J Clin Microbiol Infect Dis 2010;29(12):1465–73.
10. El Hoss S, Dussiot M, Renaud O, et al. A novel non-invasive method to measure splenic filtration function in humans. Haematologica 2018;103(10):e436–9.

11. Angay O, Friedrich M, Pinnecker J, et al. Image-based modeling and scoring of Howell-Jolly Bodies in human erythrocytes. Cytometry A 2018;93(3):305–13.
12. Corazza GR, Ginaldi L, Zoli G, et al. Howell-Jolly body counting as a measure of splenic function. A reassessment. Clin Lab Haematol 1990;12(3):269–75.
13. Lammers AJ, de Porto AP, Bennink RJ, et al. Hyposplenism: comparison of different methods for determining splenic function. Am J Hematol 2012;87(5):484–9.
14. Harrod VL, Howard TA, Zimmerman SA, et al. Quantitative analysis of Howell-Jolly bodies in children with sickle cell disease. Exp Hematol 2007;35(2):179–83.
15. William BM, Corazza GR. Hyposplenism: a comprehensive review. Part I: basic concepts and causes. Hematology 2007;12(1):1–13.
16. Rogers ZR, Wang WC, Luo Z, et al. Biomarkers of splenic function in infants with sickle cell anemia: baseline data from the BABY HUG Trial. Blood 2011;117(9): 2614–7.
17. Casper JT, Koethe S, Rodey GE, et al. A new method for studying splenic reticuloendothelial dysfunction in sickle cell disease patients and its clinical application: a brief report. Blood 1976;47(2):183–8.
18. Corazza GR, Bullen AW, Hall R, et al. Simple method of assessing splenic function in coeliac disease. Clin Sci (Lond) 1981;60(1):109–13.
19. Pearson HA, Gallagher D, Chilcote R, et al. Developmental pattern of splenic dysfunction in sickle cell disorders. Pediatrics 1985;76(3):392–7.
20. Mahlaoui N, Minard-Colin V, Picard C, et al. Isolated congenital asplenia: a French nationwide retrospective survey of 20 cases. J Pediatr 2011;158(1): 142–8, 148.e1.
21. Gilbert B, Menetrey C, Belin V, et al. Familial isolated congenital asplenia: a rare, frequently hereditary dominant condition, often detected too late as a cause of overwhelming pneumococcal sepsis. Report of a new case and review of 31 others. Eur J Pediatr 2002;161(7):368–72.
22. Bolze A, Boisson B, Bosch B, et al. Incomplete penetrance for isolated congenital asplenia in humans with mutations in translated and untranslated RPSA exons. Proc Natl Acad Sci U S A 2018;115(34):E8007–16.
23. Bolze A, Mahlaoui N, Byun M, et al. Ribosomal protein SA haploinsufficiency in humans with isolated congenital asplenia. Science 2013;340(6135):976–8.
24. Baban A, Cantarutti N, Adorisio R, et al. Long-term survival and phenotypic spectrum in heterotaxy syndrome: A 25-year follow-up experience. Int J Cardiol 2018; 268:100–5.
25. Ivemark BI. Implications of agenesis of the spleen on the pathogenesis of conotruncus anomalies in childhood; an analysis of the heart malformations in the splenic agenesis syndrome, with fourteen new cases. Acta Paediatr Suppl 1955;44(Suppl 104):7–110.
26. Thiene G, Frescura C. Asplenia and polysplenia syndromes: time of successful treatment and updated terminology. Int J Cardiol 2019;274:117–9.
27. Loomba RS, Geddes GC, Basel D, et al. Bacteremia in Patients with Heterotaxy: A Review and Implications for Management. Congenit Heart Dis 2016;11(6):537–47.
28. Friedman TC, Thomas PM, Fleisher TA, et al. Frequent occurrence of asplenism and cholelithiasis in patients with autoimmune polyglandular disease type I. Am J Med 1991;91(6):625–30.
29. Perheentupa J. Autoimmune polyendocrinopathy-candidiasis-ectodermal dystrophy. J Clin Endocrinol Metab 2006;91(8):2843–50.
30. Borsani O, Piga D, Costa S, et al. Stormorken Syndrome Caused by a p.R304W STIM1 Mutation: The First Italian Patient and a Review of the Literature. Front Neurol 2018;9:859.

31. Kulkarni S, Powles R, Treleaven J, et al. Chronic graft versus host disease is associated with long-term risk for pneumococcal infections in recipients of bone marrow transplants. Blood 2000;95(12):3683–6.
32. Corazza GR, Zoli G, Di Sabatino A, et al. A reassessment of splenic hypofunction in celiac disease. Am J Gastroenterol 1999;94(2):391–7.
33. Di Sabatino A, Rosado MM, Cazzola P, et al. Splenic hypofunction and the spectrum of autoimmune and malignant complications in celiac disease. Clin Gastroenterol Hepatol 2006;4(2):179–86.
34. Simons M, Scott-Sheldon LAJ, Risech-Neyman Y, et al. Celiac Disease and Increased Risk of Pneumococcal Infection: A Systematic Review and Meta-Analysis. Am J Med 2018;131(1):83–9.
35. Di Sabatino A, Rosado MM, Ciccocioppo R, et al. Depletion of immunoglobulin M memory B cells is associated with splenic hypofunction in inflammatory bowel disease. Am J Gastroenterol 2005;100(8):1788–95.
36. Kantso B, Simonsen J, Hoffmann S, et al. Inflammatory Bowel Disease Patients Are at Increased Risk of Invasive Pneumococcal Disease: A Nationwide Danish Cohort Study 1977-2013. Am J Gastroenterol 2015;110(11):1582–7.
37. Di Sabatino A, Aronico N, Giuffrida P, et al. Association between defective spleen function and primary eosinophilic gastrointestinal disorders. J Allergy Clin Immunol Pract 2018;6(3):1056–8.e1.
38. Giuffrida P, Aronico N, Rosselli M, et al. Defective spleen function in autoimmune gastrointestinal disorders. Intern Emerg Med 2019;15(2):225–9.
39. Dillon AM, Stein HB, English RA. Splenic atrophy in systemic lupus erythematosus. Ann Intern Med 1982;96(1):40–3.
40. Wotton CJ, Goldacre MJ. Risk of invasive pneumococcal disease in people admitted to hospital with selected immune-mediated diseases: record linkage cohort analyses. J Epidemiol Community Health 2012;66(12):1177–81.
41. Ramsahoye BH, Evely R, Mumar-Bashi W, et al. Selective IgA deficiency and hyposplenism. Clin Lab Haematol 1994;16(4):375–7.
42. Okabayashi T, Hanazaki K. Overwhelming postsplenectomy infection syndrome in adults - a clinically preventable disease. World J Gastroenterol 2008;14(2):176–9.
43. Price VE, Blanchette VS, Ford-Jones EL. The prevention and management of infections in children with asplenia or hyposplenia. Infect Dis Clin North Am 2007;21(3):697–710, viii-ix.
44. Bisharat N, Omari H, Lavi I, et al. Risk of infection and death among postsplenectomy patients. J Infect 2001;43(3):182–6.
45. Theilacker C, Ludewig K, Serr A, et al. Overwhelming Postsplenectomy Infection: A Prospective Multicenter Cohort Study. Clin Infect Dis 2016;62(7):871–8.
46. Lynch AM, Kapila R. Overwhelming postsplenectomy infection. Infect Dis Clin North Am 1996;10(4):693–707.
47. William BM, Thawani N, Sae-Tia S, et al. Hyposplenism: a comprehensive review. Part II: clinical manifestations, diagnosis, and management. Hematology 2007;12(2):89–98.
48. Spelman D, Buttery J, Daley A, et al. Guidelines for the prevention of sepsis in asplenic and hyposplenic patients. Intern Med J 2008;38(5):349–56.
49. Crary SE, Buchanan GR. Vascular complications after splenectomy for hematologic disorders. Blood 2009;114(14):2861–8.
50. Takahashi F, Uchida K, Nagaoka T, et al. Isolated congenital spleen agenesis: a rare cause of chronic thromboembolic pulmonary hypertension in an adult. Respirology 2008;13(6):913–5.

51. El-Alfy MS, El-Sayed MH. Overwhelming postsplenectomy infection: is quality of patient knowledge enough for prevention? Hematol J 2004;5(1):77–80.
52. Kim HS, Kriegel G, Aronson MD. Improving the preventive care of asplenic patients. Am J Med 2012;125(5):454–6.
53. Arnott A, Jones P, Franklin LJ, et al. A Registry for Patients With Asplenia/Hyposplenism Reduces the Risk of Infections With Encapsulated Organisms. Clin Infect Dis 2018;67(4):557–61.
54. Use of 13-valent pneumococcal conjugate vaccine and 23-valent pneumococcal polysaccharide vaccine among children aged 6-18 years with immunocompromising conditions: recommendations of the Advisory Committee on Immunization Practices (ACIP). MMWR Morb Mortal Wkly Rep 2013;62(25):521–4.
55. Use of 13-valent pneumococcal conjugate vaccine and 23-valent pneumococcal polysaccharide vaccine for adults with immunocompromising conditions: recommendations of the Advisory Committee on Immunization Practices (ACIP). MMWR Morb Mortal Wkly Rep 2012;61(40):816–9.
56. MacNeil JR, Rubin L, McNamara L, et al. Use of MenACWY-CRM vaccine in children aged 2 through 23 months at increased risk for meningococcal disease: recommendations of the Advisory Committee on Immunization Practices, 2013. MMWR Morb Mortal Wkly Rep 2014;63(24):527–30.
57. Briere EC, Rubin L, Moro PL, et al. Prevention and control of haemophilus influenzae type b disease: recommendations of the advisory committee on immunization practices (ACIP). MMWR Recomm Rep 2014;63(Rr-01):1–14.
58. Folaranmi T, Rubin L, Martin SW, et al. Use of serogroup B meningococcal vaccines in persons aged ≥10 years at increased risk for serogroup B meningococcal disease: recommendations of the Advisory Committee on Immunization Practices, 2015. MMWR Morb Mortal Wkly Rep 2015;64(22):608–12.
59. Rubin LG, Levin MJ, Ljungman P, et al. 2013 IDSA clinical practice guideline for vaccination of the immunocompromlsed host. Clin Infect Dis 2014;58(3):309–18.
60. Rubin LG, Schaffner W. Clinical practice. Care of the asplenic patient. N Engl J Med 2014;371(4):349–56.
61. Hirst C, Owusu-Ofori S. Prophylactic antibiotics for preventing pneumococcal infection in children with sickle cell disease. Cochrane Database Syst Rev 2014;(11):CD003427.
62. Kanhutu K, Jones P, Cheng AC, et al. Spleen Australia guidelines for the prevention of sepsis in patients with asplenia and hyposplenism in Australia and New Zealand. Intern Med J 2017;47(8):848–55.
63. American Academy of Pediatrics. Immunization in Special Clinical Circumstances. In: Kimberlin DW, Brady MT, Jackson MA, Long SS, editors. Red Book: 2018 Report of the Committee on Infectious Disease. 31st edition. Itasca, IL: American Academy of Pediatrics; 2018. p. 88–90.
64. Squire JD, Gardner PJ, Moutsopoulos NM, et al. Antibiotic prophylaxis for dental treatment in patients with immunodeficiency. J Allergy Clin Immunol Pract 2019; 7(3):819–23.
65. Foley PT, Kavnoudias H, Cameron PU, et al. Proximal versus distal splenic artery embolisation for blunt splenic trauma: what is the impact on splenic immune function? Cardiovasc Intervent Radiol 2015;38(5):1143–51.
66. Rodeghiero F. A critical appraisal of the evidence for the role of splenectomy in adults and children with ITP. Br J Haematol 2018;181(2):183–95.
67. Wong GK, Goldacker S, Winterhalter C, et al. Outcomes of splenectomy in patients with common variable immunodeficiency (CVID): a survey of 45 patients. Clin Exp Immunol 2013;172(1):63–72.

Hemophagocytic Lymphohistiocytosis
Lessons Learned from the Dark Side

Deepak Chellapandian, MD, MBBS

KEYWORDS

- Hemophagocytic syndrome • Secondary hemophagocytic lymphohistiocytosis
- Primary immunodeficiency • Hyperinflammation
- Flow cytometry-based primary immunodeficiency disorder screening tests
- Targeted therapy • Hematopoietic cell transplantation

KEY POINTS

- Primary hemophagocytic lymphohistiocytosis (HLH) is an inherited life-threatening hyper-inflammatory condition caused by defects in cytotoxic T lymphocytes and natural killer (NK) cells that are normally involved in mediating the control of infectious and inflammatory conditions in the immune system and tissues.
- Defects in NK cell and T cell granule-mediated cytotoxicity result in ineffective clearance of infectious agents, accumulation of antigen-presenting cells, continued stimulation and overactivation of T cells, and ultimately a cytokine storm.
- Infection, autoimmune conditions, and malignancy are important immunologic triggers for secondary HLH.
- Combining perforin expression and CD107a expression by flow cytometry has excellent diagnostic accuracy for primary HLH.

INTRODUCTION

Hemophagocytic lymphohistiocytosis (HLH) is a heterogeneous group of disorders typified by excessive activation of the immune system. It was originally named as "familial hemophagocytic reticulocytosis" in 1952 when it was first described by Farquhar and Claireaux[1] at the University of Edinburg. They recognized a constellation of signs and symptoms in a brother and sister, otherwise healthy at birth, who developed recurrent unexplained fever, bruising, pancytopenia, and hepatosplenomegaly noted at the third month of life. At autopsy, both children demonstrated hyperproliferation of histiocytes, inflammatory infiltration in the liver mostly of lymphocytes and plasma cells, many of which manifested erythrophagocytosis, and a highly reactive bone marrow.

Blood and Marrow Transplant Program, Cancer and Blood Disorders Institute, Johns Hopkins All Children's Hospital, Johns Hopkins University School of Medicine, 600 Fifth Street South, 4th Floor, St. Petersburg, FL 33701, USA
E-mail address: dchella2@jhmi.edu

Immunol Allergy Clin N Am 40 (2020) 485–497
https://doi.org/10.1016/j.iac.2020.04.003
0889-8561/20/© 2020 Elsevier Inc. All rights reserved.
immunology.theclinics.com

HLH comprises inborn defects in cytotoxic lymphocytes (particularly in natural killer [NK] cells, cytotoxic T cells [CTLs], and T-regulatory cells) that are normally involved in mediating the control of infectious and inflammatory conditions within the immune system and in other tissues.[2] In 2018, the Histiocyte Society steering committee published its consensus statement in which HLH is classified under 3 categories:

1. Primary "familial" HLH, when there is a family member affected by HLH or a known genetic defect in lymphocyte cytotoxicity
2. MAS (macrophage activation syndrome)-HLH,[3] where there is an underlying auto-immune condition triggering the pathologic inflammation
3. Secondary HLH, often associated with underlying medical conditions such as infections (eg, Epstein-Barr virus [EBV][4]), malignancy[5] (mostly lymphoid), metabolic disorders, or inherited or secondary immunodeficiencies

HLH has gained growing recognition not only in pediatric population but also increasingly in adults over the past 2 decades.

PATHOPHYSIOLOGY

Granule-mediated cytotoxic function of NK cells and CTLs is essential for clearance of viral infection and regulation and termination of the inflammatory response.[6] Defects in NK cell and CTL granule-mediated cytotoxicity result in ineffective clearance of infectious agents and defective suppression of antigen presentation. Consequently, antigen-presenting cells accumulate and continue to stimulate T cells, further escalating T cell activation and proliferation.[6] Overwhelming T cell and macrophage activation results in a cytokine storm characterized by marked elevation of cytokines, such as interferon (IFN)-γ, tumor necrosis factor (TNF)-α, interleukin (IL)-6, IL-8, IL-10, IL-12, IL-18, and macrophage colony-stimulating factor.[2] IFN-γ has been shown to play a critical role in macrophage activation and hemophagocytosis.[7,8] Elevated TNF levels lead to hypofibrinogenemia[2] and hypertriglyceridemia.[9] Gene expression studies in the peripheral blood of patients with active HLH have revealed down-regulation of genes involved in innate and adaptive immune systems, including Toll-like receptor expression and B cell and T cell function, suggesting an immunodeficiency-like state during active HLH with heightened susceptibility to infections.[10] The pathophysiology of secondary HLH is not well understood; however, finding of an HLH-like condition from repeated Toll-like receptor 9 stimulation in a murine model could explain the potential mechanism of HLH in inflammatory conditions even with normal T cell cytotoxicity.[11]

In patients with genetic changes associated with inflammasome regulation including XIAP deficiency and activating mutations in NLRC4, HLH is thought to be triggered by hyperactive macrophages and other inflammatory cells that overproduce inflammasome-dependent cytokines such as IL-18.[12] The HLH inflammasome conditions are often indistinguishable from granule-mediated cytotoxicity.

CLINICAL PRESENTATION

The clinical manifestations of HLH, either primary or secondary, are related to

1. Hyperactivation of CD8+ T-cells and macrophages
2. Hyperproliferation, ectopic migration, and tissue infiltration of these cells into various organs
3. Hypersecretion of proinflammatory cytokines, resulting in a cytokine storm and progressive tissue damage and organ dysfunction ultimately leading to death

Familial HLH (fHLH) predominantly affects infants and young children. Recent reports suggest that it can affect all age groups, from preterm neonates[13] to elderly adults.[14] With increasing awareness, HLH is more frequently diagnosed in infants, although its occurrence in neonates and older adults is under-recognized.[13,15] HLH in neonates is often misdiagnosed as sepsis and mismanaged with antimicrobials alone without concurrent anti-inflammatory medications. Acute liver failure may dominate the clinical presentation of HLH in neonates.[16] Fever is uncommon in neonates, especially those born preterm. Herpes simplex virus and enterovirus are common triggers of severe HLH in the neonatal period.[17]

Classic manifestations of HLH include high-grade unremitting fever, hepatosplenomegaly, skin rash, jaundice, bleeding, variable central nervous system (CNS) abnormalities, and laboratory findings of progressive cytopenias, coagulopathy, liver dysfunction, hyperbilirubinemia, hyperlipidemia, hyperferritinemia, hypoalbuminemia, and hyponatremia. CNS involvement occurs in 30% to 73% of HLH patients, and can include seizures, altered levels of consciousness, and brain stem symptoms, portending worse outcomes.[18] Worsening pulmonary function is an ominous sign and should suggest inadequate control of HLH and/or infection.[19]

HLH, if untreated, is potentially fatal. Interestingly, milder recurrent episodes of HLH have been noted in patients with STX11 and XIAP compared with other forms of fHLH.[20] Colitis has been reported in a significant proportion of patients with defects of STXBP2 (38%),[21] XIAP (17%),[22] and NLRC4 mutation.[23] Hypogammaglobulinemia is reported in two-thirds of patients with defects of XLP-1.[22]

"GENETIC" HEMOPHAGOCYTIC LYMPHOHISTIOCYTOSIS

In the late 1990s, the first genetic discoveries of predisposition to HLH appeared with the demonstration of pathologic variants in PRF1, LYST, and SH2D1A.[24–27] Ever since, the scope of genetic susceptibility to HLH has revolutionized the field. It is critical to make a timely distinction between the genetic HLH and the other nonhereditary HLH syndromes, as patients with genetic forms of HLH could be optimally treated by an allogeneic hematopoietic cell transplantation (HCT).

Granule-mediated CTLs function is essential for the control of infection and immune homeostasis. Perforin and granzyme B are granules within the CTLs that develop during the process of hematopoietic development that facilitates subtle degradation of the cells throughout the body and are also senescent and/or toxic to the organism.[6] Mutations in genes that encode proteins critical to the lymphocyte granule-mediated cytotoxic pathway lead to fHLH. Based on genetic etiology, fHLH has been categorized into 5 subtypes. The mutation in fHLH-1 remains unidentified, while the pathologic changes in PRF1, UNC13D, STX11, and STXBP2 are described as familial HLH-2-5,[20,28–31] respectively. HLH has been a predominant manifestation in several other genetic diseases that could be collectively called the genetic HLH diseases.[32] These diseases include certain pigmentary disorders (RAB27A, LYST and AP3B1),[25,33,34] X-linked lymphoproliferative disorders (XLP),[27] X-linked inhibitor of apoptosis (XIAP),[35] EBV-susceptibility disorders (ITK, CD27, MAGT1, CTPS1, and RASGRP1),[36–39] CDC42,[40] and activating mutation in NLRC4[12] (Table 1).

SECONDARY HEMOPHAGOCYTIC LYMPHOHISTIOCYTOSIS

Infection and malignancy are 2 common immunologic triggers for HLH that can either act alone or in concert with underlying genetic susceptibility factors.[41] Various infectious agents have been associated with HLH, with viral-associated HLH by far the

Table 1
Genetic defects associated with predisposition to hemophagocytic lymphohistiocytosis

Condition/Defective Gene	Defective Pathway/Functions
Familial HLH	
fHLH1 (unknown)	
fHLH2 (*PRF1*)	Defective CTL granule-mediated cytotoxicity
fHLH3 (*Munc 13.4*)	Defective CTL granule-mediated cytotoxicity
fHLH4 (*STX11*)	Defective CTL granule-mediated cytotoxicity
fHLH5 (*STXBP2*)	Defective CTL granule-mediated cytotoxicity
Syndromes	
Chediak Higashi syndrome (*LYST*)	Defective CTL granule-mediated cytotoxicity
Griscelli syndrome type II (*RAB27a*)	Defective CTL granule-mediated cytotoxicity
Hermansky-Pudlak syndrome type II (*AP3B1*)	Defective CTL granule-mediated cytotoxicity
EBV driven	
XLP-1 (*SH2D1A*)	SLAMR/SAP pathway; T and NK cytotoxicity and activation induced cell death
XLP-2/XIAP (*BIRC4*)	Excess apoptosis of effector cells; dysregulated NLRP3 inflammasome function
IL-2 inducible T cell kinase deficiency (*ITK*)	TCR induced calcium flux; T cell proliferation
CD27 deficiency (*CD27*)	CD27–CD70 pathway; T cell proliferation; NK cytotoxicity
XMEN (*MAGT1*)	Defective Mg++ transporter; NKG2D-dependent cytotoxicity
CD70	CD27–CD70 pathway (T cell proliferation); decreased iNKT cells; required for normal expansion and cytotoxicity of T cells
CTPS1	De novo pyrimidine synthesis; T and B cell proliferation
RASGRP1	MAPK pathway; ERK1/2, T, B cell proliferation; actin/cytoskeleton dynamics NK cytotoxicity
NLRC4	Constitutively active NLRC4 inflammasome function
CDC42	Defective formation of actin-based structures; defective proliferation, migration, and cytotoxicity; increased IL-1β and IL-18 production

most common form.[42] Herpes family viruses, including EBV, adenovirus, and cytomegalovirus (CMV), are frequent causes of infection associated HLH. Other infections influenced by geography, season, and socioeconomic status such as leishmaniasis, tick-borne illnesses, influenza, ebola, dengue, malaria and tuberculosis have been reported to be possible triggers for HLH. Almost any serious infection can trigger HLH; hence an infectious disease consultation is warranted in most HLH patients. Although infections alone can lead to secondary HLH, they are also the common trigger for overwhelming immune activation in fHLH. Hence, every attempt should be made to identify a possible genetic predisposition for HLH even in the presence of an obvious infectious trigger.

Systemic-onset juvenile idiopathic arthritis and systemic lupus erythematosus are the most common rheumatologic conditions associated with MAS.[43,44] Lymphomas, in particular T cell and NK cell lymphomas, and acute lymphoblastic leukemia have been associated with HLH.[5,45] Recently, HLH has been reported in a subset of patients with Langerhans cell histiocytosis, a form of myeloid neoplasm, who presented with multisystem disease.[46] Of note, HLH is caused by an underlying malignancy in more than 50% of the adult cases, mandating a robust evaluation of malignancy in adults presenting with HLH. HLH can occur during chemotherapy and is often associated with infection.[47] Cytokine release syndrome associated with treatment using chimeric antigen receptor (CAR)-modified T cells or bispecific T cell-engaging (BiTE) antibodies could mimic HLH.[48,49]

CONSIDERATION OF HEMOPHAGOCYTIC LYMPHOHISTIOCYTOSIS IN PRIMARY IMMUNE DEFICIENCY DISORDERS AND METABOLIC DISORDERS

HLH could be an initial presentation of several primary immunodeficiency disorders (PIDDs) (**Table 2**). In a large survey reported by Bode and colleagues,[50] 63 patients were identified with primary immunodeficiency diseases other than familial HLH, XLP, or pigmentary disorders that presented as conditions that were fulfilling current criteria for HLH. Most patients had chronic granulomatous disease (CGD) or severe combined immunodeficiency (SCID), followed by various other combined immunodeficiency disorders such as Wiskott-Aldrich syndrome, ataxia-telangiectasia, DiGeorge syndrome, and autoimmune lymphoproliferative disease syndrome (ALPS). Viruses including EBV, adenovirus, and CMV were often triggers for HLH in patients with SCID and CID, while infections such as Burkholderia cepacia, Leishmania species, and fungi triggered HLH in patients with CGD. Notably, many SCID and CGD patients presented with HLH prior to the diagnosis of SCID or CGD, highlighting the importance in considering an underlying PIDD in young patients presenting with HLH. Compared to patients with fHLH with underlying cytotoxicity defects, patients with T cell deficiencies had lower levels of soluble IL-2 receptors and higher ferritin concentrations.

Table 2 Selected primary immunodeficiency disorders and inborn error of metabolism complicated by hemophagocytic lymphohistiocytosis	
Primary Immunodeficiency Disorders	**Inborn Error of Metabolism**
Severe combined immune deficiency	Lysinuric protein intolerance
Chronic granulomatous disease	Galactosemia
CTLA4 haploinsufficiency	Gaucher disease
STAT1 gain of function	Pearson syndrome
STAT3	Biotinidase deficiency
APDS	Wolman disease
GATA2	Niemann–Pick disease
NEMO	Long-chain 3-hydroxyacyl-CoA dehydrogenase
DOCK8	(LCHAD) deficiency
ALPS	Methylmalonic acidemia
Wiskott-Aldrich syndrome	
Ataxia-Telangiectasia	
ORAI-1 deficiency	
Tumor necrosis factor receptor-associated periodic syndrome (TRAPS)	
Familial Mediterranean fever (FMF)	

Another large single center reported the identification of primary immune deficiencies in 14 out of 47 pediatric patients (30%) with HLH who lacked a genetic HLH disease.[51] The high percentage of PIDD patients found in this cohort underscores the importance of whole-exome sequencing or large PIDD panel testing in patients with HLH without identifiable linkage to HLH causing disease. Several inborn errors of metabolism can also present with HLH, in particular, lysinuric protein intolerance.[52] The exact mechanism is not well understood; however, the accumulation of nondegraded substrates in macrophages may potentially lead to inflammasome activation, thereby triggering uncontrolled activation of macrophages, and ultimately development of HLH.

DIAGNOSTIC WORK-UP

The Histiocyte Society established a set of clinical and laboratory criteria to help formalize the diagnosis of HLH. In order to fit the diagnosis of HLH, a patient needs to have a genetic diagnosis or meet at least 5 of 8 diagnostic criteria put forth by the Histiocyte Society[53] (**Box 1**). Although intended for the conduct of clinical trials, these diagnostic criteria have been widely used for diagnosing and treating patients regardless of their participation in clinical trial. However, it should be noted that these diagnostic criteria do not reflect all of the typical clinical or laboratory features of patients with HLH, many of which are helpful in making the diagnosis. For example, transaminitis is not among the 8 diagnostic criteria; however, patients with HLH almost always present with inflammation of liver, which could range from mild transaminitis to fulminant liver failure. Hence a diagnosis of HLH in the absence of transaminitis should be considered unusual.

Ferritin, an acute-phase reactant secreted by macrophages, is widely used as a screening test for HLH/MAS. Ferritin greater than 10,000 mg/L has been reported to be highly specific and diagnostic of HLH.[54] Soluble IL-2 receptor (soluble CD25), a marker of activated T lymphocytes, is a useful screening tool in diagnosis and for monitoring of patients with HLH. Soluble CD163, a marker of monocyte/macrophage

---

Box 1

Diagnostic Criteria for hemophagocytic lymphohistiocytosis

The diagnosis of HLH can be established if one of either 1 or 2 below is fulfilled:
1. A molecular diagnosis consistent with HLH is made
2. Diagnostic criteria for HLH are fulfilled (5 of the 8 criteria below)
    Fever
    Splenomegaly
    Cytopenias (affecting 2 of the 3 lineages in the peripheral blood):
        Hemoglobin < 90 g/L (in infants <4 wk of age, hemoglobin <100 g/L)
        Platelets less than $100 \times 10^9/L$
        Neutrophils less than $1.0 \times 10^9/L$
    Hypertriglyceridemia and/or hypofibrinogenemia:
        Fasting triglycerides ≥ 3.0 mmol/L (ie, ≥ 265 mg/dL)
        Fibrinogen ≤ 1.5 g/L
    Hemophagocytosis in bone marrow or spleen or lymph nodes
    Low or absent NK cell activity (according to local laboratory reference)
    Ferritin ≥ 500 mg/L
    Soluble IL-2 receptor (ie, soluble CD25) ≥ 2400 U/mL

From Henter JI, Horne A, Aricó M, et al. HLH-2004: diagnostic and therapeutic guidelines for hemophagocytic lymphohistiocytosis. Pediatr Blood Cancer 2007;48(2):124-31; with permission.

activation, also has been reported to be useful in diagnosing HLH.[55] Elevations of multiple proinflammatory cytokines are seen in patients with HLH, and markedly elevated levels of IFN-γ, and IL-10 have been identified as helpful markers in diagnosing HLH.[56] CXCL-9, which indicates IFN-γ pathway activity, and IL-18, a marker of inflammasome activation are being increasingly used in diagnosing hyperinflammatory conditions. The ratio of IL-18 to CXCL9 has been used to differentiate patients with rheumatologic diseases and macrophage activation syndrome from patients with HLH with ratios less than 2.3 favoring fHLH over MAS.[57]

Prompt evaluation for infection and malignancies should be performed in all patients suspected for HLH, including laboratory studies, diagnostic images, bone marrow studies, and biopsy of clinically suspicious findings. Of note, bone marrow aspirate has a sensitivity of only 60%.[58] Hence a negative bone marrow analysis should not preclude initiation of therapy if there is high clinical suspicion and laboratory evidence of HLH. Sensitivity of bone marrow analysis could be improved by the addition of CD163 immunohistochemistry.[59] Robust infectious and oncological assessment is mandatory for adult cases, as most HLH is reactive and secondary to malignancy, followed by infections.

Several reliable flow cytometry-based PIDD screening tests are available to screen for causes of fHLH.[60] Quantitative assessment of intracellular perforin, signaling lymphocyte-activating molecule–associated protein and XIAP, is available clinically and has a sensitivity of greater than 80%.[60] NK cell cytotoxicity is more time consuming and might not be depressed in all patients. Surface expression of CD107a on NK cells and CTLs is used to measure the integrity of the lymphocyte granule-mediated cytotoxicity pathway. CD107a is found within the membranes of cytotoxic granules, and is often expressed on the surface of the cell with degranulation; the increase can be measured by flow cytometry. The NK cell CD107a assay offers greater than 90% sensitivity, and, unlike the NK cell cytotoxicity assay, does not appear to be greatly influenced by steroid use. Combining perforin expression and CD107a expression by flow cytometry has excellent diagnostic accuracy for primary HLH.[61]

Genetic diagnostic testing using next-generation sequencing panels or whole-exome sequencing should be sent for all patients suspected of fHLH. Targeted sequencing may be considered in select patients such as family history of a specific genetic defect, or a positive screening test highly suggestive of a single likely gene (ie, absent perforin expression). For patients with negative screening work-up, other differential diagnoses such as PIDDs, metabolic diseases, occult infections, and malignancies should be strongly considered.

TREATMENT

The fundamental principle of management of HLH includes a short-term strategy to control the hyperinflammatory state and a long-term strategy aimed at definitively correcting the underlying genetic defect by using an allogenic HCT.

The control of hyperinflammatory state is achieved using chemotherapeutic agents, immunosuppressants, and targeted biologic agents, and aims to eliminate activated T cells and macrophages, and dampen the cytokine storm.

A commonly used treatment approach consists of 8-week course of dexamethasone and etoposide based on the experiences of the Histiocyte Society HLH-94 protocol and afterward considering HCT in selected cases.[62] Patients with central nervous system involvement received additional targeted intrathecal treatment with methotrexate and steroid therapy. With this protocol, the remission induction rate was 71%, and 5-year post-HCT survival probability was 54% +/− 6%.[63] Transplantation outcomes were better in patients with adequately controlled HLH activity before HCT.[63] Upfront addition of cyclosporine to dexamethasone and etoposide did not improve the outcome of patients in HLH-2004 study.[64] A single-center study from France showed a promising remission rate of 70% with a chemotherapy-sparing approach consisting of steroids, antithymocyte globulin (ATG), and cyclosporin.[65]

Until recently, there was no second line pretransplant treatment for HLH refractory to etoposide-based therapy. Alemtuzumab, a monoclonal antibody to CD52, reportedly induced partial response in 64% of treated patients.[66] The transplantation outcomes are better in patients with adequately controlled HLH activity prior to HCT. Therefore, in patients who are refractory to etoposide-containing HLH-94–based induction therapy, alemtuzumab might be useful salvage therapy for better disease control before proceeding to HCT. Alemtuzumab is currently being evaluated in a clinical trial that enrolls subjects affected by primary HLH (NCT02472054).

Unlike with fHLH, there is no consensus on management of secondary HLH. In MAS-HLH, therapy with pulsed steroids and/or cyclosporine has demonstrated a good response.[67] Various other[68,69] targeted therapies, including alemtuzumab, infliximab, etanercept, and daclizumab, have been identified to be useful. Rituximab, a CD20 monoclonal antibody, when used in conjunction with conventional HLH-directed therapy in EBV-triggered HLH, has been shown to improve clinical symptoms, viral load, and inflammation.[4] In both primary and secondary HLH, management of associated infection is critical for resolving HLH. Moreover, in infection-associated HLH, management of infection alone is often not sufficient for clinical improvement; some form of immunosuppressive/immunomodulatory therapy might be necessary to manage the accompanying hyperinflammatory state.[42]

Chinn and colleagues[51] reported that in 48 patients with HLH, whole-exome sequencing analysis was able to identify a genetic diagnosis of primary immune deficiency in 30% patients. This study offered an opportunity to understand the exact underlying molecular mechanism of disease and target treatment. For example, in a patient diagnosed with STAT3 GOF, JAK inhibition and IL-6 blockade therapy were successful in reversing the clinical and laboratory manifestations of HLH.[70] IFN-γ has been shown in several in vitro and in vivo studies as a major driver of pathologic inflammation in HLH.[8] Emapalumab, a monoclonal antibody against IFN-γ, has been recently approved by the US Food and Drug Administration (FDA) for use in patients with adult or pediatric primary HLH that is refractory, recurrent, or progressive or intolerant to conventional HLH therapy.[71,72] Of note, the initial study did not include adult patients. Emapalumab is given as an intravenous infusion every 3 to 4 days; it is initiated at a dose of 1 mg/kg concomitant with dexamethasone (5–10 mg/m² per day) and increased up to 10 mg/kg based on clinical response assessed by clinical and laboratory markers. The JAK/STAT pathway lies downstream of several cytokines that are elevated in HLH and could represent an attractive therapeutic target to abrogate the signaling of multiple cytokine pathways. JAK/STAT inhibition with ruxolitinib, a JAK1/2 inhibitor, has been shown to decrease anemia, thrombocytopenia, organomegaly, tissue damage, and cytokine levels in the $Prf1^{-/-}$ murine model of HLH.[73,74] A phase I trial evaluating ruxolitinib for patients with HLH is currently recruiting patients (NCT02400463). A clinical trial is currently evaluating recombinant human IL-18 binding protein (tadekinig alfa) for patients with inflammasome activation and high IL-18 levels such as patients with NLRC4 mutations[75] or XIAP deficiency (NCT03113760).

Although primary HLH can be controlled by immunochemotherapy, HCT is ultimately required as a curative therapy. Historical data suggest poor overall survival (approximately 50%) of genetic forms of HLH proceeding to HCT, mostly related to regimen-related toxicity and infections.[63,76] Patients with XIAP deficiency are likely susceptible to complications of graft versus host disease.[77] Recently, Allen and colleagues[78] showed reduced morbidity and mortality associated with reduced-intensity regimens using melphalan, fludarabine, and intermediate-timing alemtuzumab, however up to 61% of the patients required a second intervention using donor lymphocyte infusion (DLI) and/or a second HCT. There is growing experience with using reduced toxicity sub myeloablative conditioning approaches for HLH. HLA typing and initiation of donor search should be done promptly as soon as a genetic form of HLH is suspected in a patient.

SUMMARY

HLH is a potentially fatal disorder of immune regulation that can present across all age groups. Significant advances have been made in the past 2 decades with regards to understanding of genetic forms of HLH, with significant gains in diagnostic modalities, treatment, and transplant experience. Secondary causes such as infectious diseases, autoimmune disease, and malignancy should be suspected when evaluating for HLH, so that disease-specific treatment can be given promptly.

Despite significant progress in outcome, front-line treatment and HCT procedures still require improvement to further reduce mortality and late sequalae of this devastating condition. Advanced genetic testing, new targeted therapeutic agents, optimization of conditioning regimens, and graft manipulation strategies for HCT may potentially overcome these challenges.

DISCLOSURE

This work is supported by Johns Hopkins All Children's Foundation Institutional Research Grant Program to D. Chellapandian.

Conflict of Interest statement: There are no conflicts of interest to report.

REFERENCES

1. Farquhar JW, Claireaux AE. Familial haemophagocytic reticulosis. Arch Dis Child 1952;27(136):519–25.
2. Henter JI, Elinder G, Soder O, et al. Hypercytokinemia in familial hemophagocytic lymphohistiocytosis. Blood 1991;78(11):2918–22.
3. Grom AA. Macrophage activation syndrome and reactive hemophagocytic lymphohistiocytosis: the same entities? Curr Opin Rheumatol 2003;15(5):587–90.
4. Chellapandian D, Das R, Zelley K, et al. Treatment of Epstein Barr virus-induced haemophagocytic lymphohistiocytosis with rituximab-containing chemo-immunotherapeutic regimens. Br J Haematol 2013;162(3):376–82.
5. Lehmberg K, Sprekels B, Nichols KE, et al. Malignancy-associated haemophagocytic lymphohistiocytosis in children and adolescents. Br J Haematol 2015; 170(4):539–49.
6. Lykens JE, Terrell CE, Zoller EE, et al. Perforin is a critical physiologic regulator of T-cell activation. Blood 2011;118(3):618–26.
7. Zoller EE, Lykens JE, Terrell CE, et al. Hemophagocytosis causes a consumptive anemia of inflammation. J Exp Med 2011;208(6):1203–14.
8. Jordan MB, Hildeman D, Kappler J, et al. An animal model of hemophagocytic lymphohistiocytosis (HLH): CD8+ T cells and interferon gamma are essential for the disorder. Blood 2004;104(3):735–43.

9. Henter JI, Carlson LA, Soder O, et al. Lipoprotein alterations and plasma lipoprotein lipase reduction in famillal hemophagocytic lymphohistiocytosis. Acta Paediatr Scand 1991;80(6–7):675–81.

10. Sumegi J, Barnes MG, Nestheide SV, et al. Gene expression profiling of peripheral blood mononuclear cells from children with active hemophagocytic lymphohistiocytosis. Blood 2011;117(15):e151–60.

11. Behrens EM, Canna SW, Slade K, et al. Repeated TLR9 stimulation results in macrophage activation syndrome-like disease in mice. J Clin Invest 2011; 121(6):2264–77.

12. Canna SW, de Jesus AA, Gouni S, et al. An activating NLRC4 inflammasome mutation causes autoinflammation with recurrent macrophage activation syndrome. Nat Genet 2014;46(10):1140–6.

13. Suzuki N, Morimoto A, Ohga S, et al. Characteristics of hemophagocytic lymphohistiocytosis in neonates: a nationwide survey in Japan. J Pediatr 2009;155(2): 235–8.e1.

14. Tabata R, Tabata C, Terada M, et al. Hemophagocytic syndrome in elderly patients with underlying autoimmune diseases. Clin Rheumatol 2009;28(4):461–4.

15. Raschke RA, Garcia-Orr R. Hemophagocytic lymphohistiocytosis: a potentially underrecognized association with systemic inflammatory response syndrome, severe sepsis, and septic shock in adults. Chest 2011;140(4):933–8.

16. Amir AZ, Ling SC, Naqvi A, et al. Liver transplantation for children with acute liver failure associated with secondary hemophagocytic lymphohistiocytosis. Liver Transpl 2016;22(9):1245–53.

17. Whaley BF. Familial hemophagocytic lymphohistiocytosis in the neonate. Adv Neonatal Care 2011;11(2):101–7.

18. Horne A, Wickstrom R, Jordan MB, et al. How to treat involvement of the central nervous system in hemophagocytic lymphohistiocytosis? Curr Treat Options Neurol 2017;19(1):3.

19. Fitzgerald NE, MacClain KL. Imaging characteristics of hemophagocytic lymphohistiocytosis. Pediatr Radiol 2003;33(6):392–401.

20. zur Stadt U, Schmidt S, Kasper B, et al. Linkage of familial hemophagocytic lymphohistiocytosis (FHL) type-4 to chromosome 6q24 and identification of mutations in syntaxin 11. Hum Mol Genet 2005;14(6):827–34.

21. Pagel J, Beutel K, Lehmberg K, et al. Distinct mutations in STXBP2 are associated with variable clinical presentations in patients with familial hemophagocytic lymphohistiocytosis type 5 (FHL5). Blood 2012;119(25):6016–24.

22. Pachlopnik Schmid J, Canioni D, Moshous D, et al. Clinical similarities and differences of patients with X-linked lymphoproliferative syndrome type 1 (XLP-1/SAP deficiency) versus type 2 (XLP-2/XIAP deficiency). Blood 2011;117(5):1522–9.

23. Romberg N, Vogel TP, Canna SW. NLRC4 inflammasomopathies. Curr Opin Allergy Clin Immunol 2017;17(6):398–404.

24. Stepp SE, Dufourcq-Lagelouse R, Le Deist F, et al. Perforin gene defects in familial hemophagocytic lymphohistiocytosis. Science 1999;286(5446):1957–9.

25. Barbosa MD, Nguyen QA, Tchernev VT, et al. Identification of the homologous beige and Chediak-Higashi syndrome genes. Nature 1996;382(6588):262–5.

26. Sayos J, Wu C, Morra M, et al. The X-linked lymphoproliferative-disease gene product SAP regulates signals induced through the co-receptor SLAM. Nature 1998;395(6701):462–9.

27. Nichols KE, Harkin DP, Levitz S, et al. Inactivating mutations in an SH2 domain-encoding gene in X-linked lymphoproliferative syndrome. Proc Natl Acad Sci U S A 1998;95(23):13765–70.

28. Janka GE, Schneider EM. Modern management of children with haemophagocytic lymphohistiocytosis. Br J Haematol 2004;124(1):4–14.
29. Dufourcq-Lagelouse R, Jabado N, Le Deist F, et al. Linkage of familial hemophagocytic lymphohistiocytosis to 10q21-22 and evidence for heterogeneity. Am J Hum Genet 1999;64(1):172–9.
30. Feldmann J, Callebaut I, Raposo G, et al. Munc13-4 is essential for cytolytic granules fusion and is mutated in a form of familial hemophagocytic lymphohistiocytosis (FHL3). Cell 2003;115(4):461–73.
31. zur Stadt U, Rohr J, Seifert W, et al. Familial hemophagocytic lymphohistiocytosis type 5 (FHL-5) is caused by mutations in Munc18-2 and impaired binding to syntaxin 11. Am J Hum Genet 2009;85(4):482–92.
32. Sepulveda FE, de Saint Basile G. Hemophagocytic syndrome: primary forms and predisposing conditions. Curr Opin Immunol 2017;49:20–6.
33. Enders A, Zieger B, Schwarz K, et al. Lethal hemophagocytic lymphohistiocytosis in Hermansky-Pudlak syndrome type II. Blood 2006;108(1):81–7.
34. Menasche G, Pastural E, Feldmann J, et al. Mutations in RAB27A cause Griscelli syndrome associated with haemophagocytic syndrome. Nat Genet 2000;25(2):173–6.
35. Marsh RA, Madden L, Kitchen BJ, et al. XIAP deficiency: a unique primary immunodeficiency best classified as X-linked familial hemophagocytic lymphohistiocytosis and not as X-linked lymphoproliferative disease. Blood 2010;116(7):1079–82.
36. Stepensky P, Weintraub M, Yanir A, et al. IL-2-inducible T-cell kinase deficiency: clinical presentation and therapeutic approach. Haematologica 2011;96(3):472–6.
37. van Montfrans JM, Hoepelman AI, Otto S, et al. CD27 deficiency is associated with combined immunodeficiency and persistent symptomatic EBV viremia. J Allergy Clin Immunol 2012;129(3):787–93.e6.
38. Li FY, Chaigne-Delalande B, Kanellopoulou C, et al. Second messenger role for Mg2+ revealed by human T-cell immunodeficiency. Nature 2011;475(7357):471–6.
39. Latour S, Winter S. Inherited immunodeficiencies with high predisposition to epstein-barr virus-driven lymphoproliferative diseases. Front Immunol 2018;9:1103.
40. Lam MT, Coppola S, Krumbach OHF, et al. A novel disorder involving dyshematopoiesis, inflammation, and HLH due to aberrant CDC42 function. J Exp Med 2019;216(12):2778–99.
41. Chesshyre E, Ramanan AV, Roderick MR. Hemophagocytic lymphohistiocytosis and infections: an update. Pediatr Infect Dis J 2019;38(3):e54–6.
42. Rouphael NG, Talati NJ, Vaughan C, et al. Infections associated with haemophagocytic syndrome. Lancet Infect Dis 2007;7(12):814–22.
43. Ravelli A, Davi S, Minoia F, et al. Macrophage Activation Syndrome. Hematol Oncol Clin North Am 2015;29(5):927–41.
44. Liu AC, Yang Y, Li MT, et al. Macrophage activation syndrome in systemic lupus erythematosus: a multicenter, case-control study in China. Clin Rheumatol 2018;37(1):93–100.
45. O'Brien MM, Lee-Kim Y, George TI, et al. Precursor B-cell acute lymphoblastic leukemia presenting with hemophagocytic lymphohistiocytosis. Pediatr Blood Cancer 2008;50(2):381–3.
46. Chellapandian, et al. Cancer 2019;125(6):963–71.

47. Parikh SA, Kapoor P, Letendre L, et al. Prognostic factors and outcomes of adults with hemophagocytic lymphohistiocytosis. Mayo Clin Proc 2014;89(4):484–92.

48. Teachey DT, Rheingold SR, Maude SL, et al. Cytokine release syndrome after blinatumomab treatment related to abnormal macrophage activation and ameliorated with cytokine-directed therapy. Blood 2013;121(26):5154–7.

49. Frey N, Porter D. Cytokine release syndrome with chimeric antigen receptor T cell therapy. Biol Blood Marrow Transplant 2019;25(4):e123–7.

50. Bode SF, Ammann S, Al-Herz W, et al. The syndrome of hemophagocytic lymphohistiocytosis in primary immunodeficiencies: implications for differential diagnosis and pathogenesis. Haematologica 2015;100(7):978–88.

51. Chinn IK, Eckstein OS, Peckham-Gregory EC, et al. Genetic and mechanistic diversity in pediatric hemophagocytic lymphohistiocytosis. Blood 2018;132(1): 89–100.

52. Duval M, Fenneteau O, Doireau V, et al. Intermittent hemophagocytic lymphohistiocytosis is a regular feature of lysinuric protein intolerance. J Pediatr 1999; 134(2):236–9.

53. Henter JI, Horne A, Arico M, et al. HLH-2004: diagnostic and therapeutic guidelines for hemophagocytic lymphohistiocytosis. Pediatr Blood Cancer 2007;48(2): 124–31.

54. Allen CE, Yu X, Kozinetz CA, et al. Highly elevated ferritin levels and the diagnosis of hemophagocytic lymphohistiocytosis. Pediatr Blood Cancer 2008;50(6): 1227–35.

55. Bleesing J, Prada A, Siegel DM, et al. The diagnostic significance of soluble CD163 and soluble interleukin-2 receptor alpha-chain in macrophage activation syndrome and untreated new-onset systemic juvenile idiopathic arthritis. Arthritis Rheum 2007;56(3):965–71.

56. Xu XJ, Tang YM, Song H, et al. Diagnostic accuracy of a specific cytokine pattern in hemophagocytic lymphohistiocytosis in children. J Pediatr 2012;160(6): 984–90.e1.

57. Weiss ES, Girard-Guyonvarc'h C, Holzinger D, et al. Interleukin-18 diagnostically distinguishes and pathogenically promotes human and murine macrophage activation syndrome. Blood 2018;131(13):1442–55.

58. Gupta A, Weitzman S, Abdelhaleem M. The role of hemophagocytosis in bone marrow aspirates in the diagnosis of hemophagocytic lymphohistiocytosis. Pediatr Blood Cancer 2008;50(2):192–4.

59. Behrens EM, Beukelman T, Paessler M, et al. Occult macrophage activation syndrome in patients with systemic juvenile idiopathic arthritis. J Rheumatol 2007; 34(5):1133–8.

60. Johnson TS, Villanueva J, Filipovich AH, et al. Contemporary diagnostic methods for hemophagocytic lymphohistiocytic disorders. J Immunol Methods 2011; 364(1–2):1–13.

61. Rubin TS, Zhang K, Gifford C, et al. Perforin and CD107a testing are superior to NK cell function testing for screening patients for genetic HLH. Blood 2017; 129(22):2993–9.

62. Ehl S, Astigarraga I, von Bahr Greenwood T, et al. Recommendations for the use of etoposide-based therapy and bone marrow transplantation for the treatment of HLH: consensus statements by the HLH Steering Committee of the Histiocyte Society. J Allergy Clin Immunol Pract 2018;6(5):1508–17.

63. Trottestam H, Horne A, Arico M, et al. Chemoimmunotherapy for hemophagocytic lymphohistiocytosis: long-term results of the HLH-94 treatment protocol. Blood 2011;118(17):4577–84.

64. Bergsten E, Horne A, Arico M, et al. Confirmed efficacy of etoposide and dexa-methasone in HLH treatment: long-term results of the cooperative HLH-2004 study. Blood 2017;130(25):2728–38.

65. Mahlaoui N, Ouachee-Chardin M, de Saint Basile G, et al. Immunotherapy of fa-milial hemophagocytic lymphohistiocytosis with antithymocyte globulins: a single-center retrospective report of 38 patients. Pediatrics 2007;120(3):e622–8.

66. Marsh RA, Allen CE, McClain KL, et al. Salvage therapy of refractory hemopha-gocytic lymphohistiocytosis with alemtuzumab. Pediatr Blood Cancer 2013; 60(1):101–9.

67. Stephan JL, Kone-Paut I, Galambrun C, et al. Reactive haemophagocytic syn-drome in children with inflammatory disorders. A retrospective study of 24 pa-tients. Rheumatology (Oxford) 2001;40(11):1285–92.

68. Grom AA, Horne A, De Benedetti F. Macrophage activation syndrome in the era of biologic therapy. Nat Rev Rheumatol 2016;12(5):259–68.

69. Schulert GS, Minoia F, Bohnsack J, et al. Effect of biologic therapy on clinical and laboratory features of macrophage activation syndrome associated with systemic juvenile idiopathic arthritis. Arthritis Care Res (Hoboken) 2018;70(3):409–19.

70. Forbes LR, Vogel TP, Cooper MA, et al. Jakinibs for the treatment of immune dys-regulation in patients with gain-of-function signal transducer and activator of tran-scription 1 (STAT1) or STAT3 mutations. J Allergy Clin Immunol 2018;142(5): 1665–9.

71. Al-Salama ZT. Emapalumab: first global approval. Drugs 2019;79(1):99–103.

72. Vallurupalli M, Berliner N. Emapalumab for the treatment of relapsed/refractory hemophagocytic lymphohistiocytosis. Blood 2019;134(21):1783–6.

73. Das R, Guan P, Sprague L, et al. Janus kinase inhibition lessens inflammation and ameliorates disease in murine models of hemophagocytic lymphohistiocytosis. Blood 2016;127(13):1666–75.

74. Albeituni S, Verblst KC, Tedrick PE, et al. Mechanisms of action of ruxolitinib in murine models of hemophagocytic lymphohistiocytosis. Blood 2019;134(2): 147–59.

75. Canna SW, Girard C, Malle L, et al. Life-threatening NLRC4-associated hyperin-flammation successfully treated with IL-18 inhibition. J Allergy Clin Immunol 2017; 139(5):1698–701.

76. Marsh RA, Jordan MB, Filipovich AH. Reduced-intensity conditioning haemato-poietic cell transplantation for haemophagocytic lymphohistiocytosis: an impor-tant step forward. Br J Haematol 2011;154(5):556–63.

77. Muller N, Fischer JC, Yabal M, et al. XIAP deficiency in hematopoietic recipient cells drives donor T-cell activation and GvHD in mice. Eur J Immunol 2019; 49(3):504–7.

78. Allen CE, Marsh R, Dawson P, et al. Reduced-intensity conditioning for hemato-poietic cell transplant for HLH and primary immune deficiencies. Blood 2018; 132(13):1438–51.

Diagnosis and management of Specific Antibody Deficiency

Elena E. Perez, MD, PhD[a],*, Mark Ballow, MD[b]

KEYWORDS

- Specific antibody deficiency • Antibody deficiency • Diagnosis
- Immunoglobulin replacement therapy • Pneumococcal vaccines • PCV13 • PPSV23
- Primary immunodeficiency

KEY POINTS

- Specific antibody deficiency is a primary antibody deficiency characterized by normal levels of immunoglobulins and subclasses, recurrent sinopulmonary infections, and poor response to polysaccharide antigens after vaccination.
- The clinical diagnosis can be challenging owing to variations of immune response with age, potential comorbid conditions, and interpretation of immune response to pneumococcal serotypes.
- Initial management may involve optimizing treatment of any coexisting allergic conditions and prophylactic antibiotics. Immune globulin replacement therapy is used in select patients.
- Guidelines exist for the interpretation of diagnostic vaccine responses, but may change over time. Several phenotypes have been defined, which can assist the clinician in management decisions regarding immune globulin replacement therapy.

INTRODUCTION

Specific antibody deficiency (SAD) is a primary immunodeficiency disease (PIDD) associated with recurrent respiratory bacterial infections and characterized by normal total IgG, IgG subclasses, IgA, and IgM levels, but with recurrent infection and diminished antibody responses to polysaccharide antigens after vaccination.[1–3] SAD is recognized by the International Union of Immunology Societies as a PIDD of unknown genetic cause that affects antibody production.[4] The term SAD refers to impaired

This article is adapted from Perez E, Bonilla FA, Orange JS, et al. Specific Antibody Deficiency: Controversies in Diagnosis and Management. Front Immunol 2017;8:586.
[a] Allergy Associates of the Palm Beaches, 840 US Highway 1, Suite 235, North Palm Beach, FL 33408, USA; [b] Department of Pediatrics, Division of Allergy and Immunology, All Children's Research Institute, University of South Florida, Johns Hopkins Children's Hospital, 140 7th Avenue South, CRI 4008, St Petersburg, FL 33701, USA
* Corresponding author.
E-mail address: eperez@pballergy.com

Immunol Allergy Clin N Am 40 (2020) 499–510
https://doi.org/10.1016/j.iac.2020.03.005
0889-8561/20/© 2020 Elsevier Inc. All rights reserved.

immunology.theclinics.com

polysaccharide vaccine responsiveness with completely normal Ig isotype levels.[5,6] Some healthy infants under 2 years of age cannot yet mount a robust response to pure unconjugated polysaccharide antigens such as *Streptococcus pneumoniae* polysaccharide and *Haemophilus influenzae* type b capsular polysaccharide. Therefore, the diagnosis of SAD should not be made until after the age of 2 years.[2,5–8]

Data on the prevalence of SAD is variable owing to changes in the definition of SAD over time, differences in study populations, and the specific criteria used to define antibody responsiveness to polysaccharide antigens.[1] SAD has been estimated to be the eighth most commonly identified PIDD globally.[9] Studies estimate the prevalence of SAD to be between 6% and 23% in children evaluated for recurrent infections,[5,10–12] between 11.6% and 24% in adults with chronic rhinosinusitis,[13–15] and approximately 8% in adults with recurrent pneumonia.[16]

The genetic cause of SAD is unknown, but decreased numbers of switched memory B cells, which may play a key role in the protection against infection with polysaccharide-encapsulated bacteria, have been reported in patients with SAD.[17] Patients with SAD are highly susceptible to severe respiratory tract infections with encapsulated bacteria, and SAD is one of the most commonly identified immune disorders in patients presenting with recurrent sinopulmonary infections.[2,14]

DIAGNOSIS

Patients with antibody deficiencies including SAD typically present with recurrent upper and lower respiratory tract infections, otitis media, and sinusitis.[1,18] Asthma and rhinitis are common in children with SAD.[1] Poor antibody response to polysaccharide antigens may also be found in other well-established PIDDs including Wiskott-Aldrich syndrome, partial DiGeorge syndrome,[18] and nuclear factor-κB essential modulator deficiency.[19] SAD can present with infections similarly to common variable immune deficiency (CVID), but the main diagnostic difference is that SAD has normal total immune globulin levels whereas CVID includes hypogammaglobulinemia and low IgA and/or IgM. SAD is generally less severe than CVID and without the various comorbid conditions of CVID.[20,21] The definition of SAD from the European Society for Immunodeficiencies (ESID) and the US practice parameters are in general agreement but have some differences (**Table 1**)[3,6,20] The ESID definition describes the defect in polysaccharide responsiveness as profound, requires the exclusion of underlying T-cell defects, and does not take into account B-cell number or patient age, whereas the US 2015 practice parameters include normal B-cell numbers and age greater than 2 years as criteria. Class switched memory B-cell percentage may be an indicator of clinical complications associated with SAD (and also CVID),[17] but this factor is not part of the clinical definition. Given that the prevalence of atopy is increased in SAD,[1] and that allergic comorbidities can predispose to infections, the diagnosis of SAD may be difficult in the context of uncontrolled allergies.

Assessing Antibody Response to the Pneumococcal Polysaccharide Vaccine

Assessment of a patient's antibody responses to vaccines is used as a surrogate marker for B-cell function in clinical immunology. The response to conjugated vaccines tests the capacity to form specific antibodies using the T-cell–dependent pathway, whereas the response to polysaccharide vaccines tests the capacity to form antibodies using the T-cell–independent pathway. Pneumococcal vaccines stimulate production of serotype specific IgG to protect against the gram-positive cocci *S pneumoniae*.[6] In the United States, the Centers for Disease Control and Prevention recommend the 13-valent pneumococcal conjugate vaccine and the 23-valent

Table 1 ESID and US practice parameters for the diagnosis of SAD		
	SAD	
	ESID Criteria[3]	US Practice Parameters[6]
Clinical presentation	Recurrent or severe bacterial infections	Recurrent respiratory tract infections
Antibody levels	Normal IgG, IgA, and IgM and IgG subclasses	
Response to vaccines	Profound alteration of the antibody responses to polysaccharide vaccine	Impaired response to pneumococcal capsular polysaccharide
B cells	Not considered	Normal B-cell levels
T cells	Exclusion of T-cell defect	Not considered
Other diagnostic criteria	None	Patients older than 2 y

pneumococcal polysaccharide vaccine (PPSV23) for adults at age 65 or in the presence of specific high-risk conditions, and a series of 13-valent pneumococcal conjugate vaccinations for children under 2 years of age.[22,23] Indications for the vaccines depend on age, previous vaccinations, and the presence of high-risk conditions, including congenital immunodeficiency.[22]

The clinical response to pneumococcal vaccines is determined by measuring the levels of serotype-specific IgG against serotypes included in the vaccine. Currently, this response is accomplished by multiplex bead immunoassay or enzyme-linked immunosorbent assay.[24–26] In the past, radioimmunoassay was used, but this method does not differentiate between antibody responses of different Ig isotypes.[27] Owing to a lack of controlled clinical studies and the absence of a standardized definition of an insufficient pneumococcal polysaccharide antibody response, the criteria for diagnosis of SAD have changed over the years. The most recent working group consensus was published in 2012.[28] The definition of a protective titer is not uniform and may vary depending on the nature of the vaccine.[6,28,29] For example, in small studies, a serotype-specific level of 1.3 μg/mL has been considered protective with respect to invasive disease after polysaccharide immunization,[28,30] whereas other studies showed that levels of 0.35 μg/mL were considered protective against invasive pneumococcal infections after immunization with a conjugate pneumococcal vaccine.[31] An adequate response to immunization was previously defined as at least a 4-fold increase in antibody levels over baseline for a given serotype.[29,32] However, this criterion is no longer preferred because evidence suggests that patients with high baseline titers may not develop a 4-fold increase in titers after vaccination[33]; furthermore, a meta-analysis of antipneumococcal antibody responses in healthy individuals, showed that the ratios of prevaccination to postvaccination titers varied widely and depended on the particular serotype and the baseline level of antibody.[30] One current recommendation is to accept a 2-fold response if the baseline level is 1.3 μg/mL or greater.[28]

Determining the precise number of pneumococcal serotypes needed for a normal response is a problem complicated by the different pneumococcal vaccines used. PPSV23, a pure polysaccharide vaccine that induces a T-cell–independent antibody response, immunizes against 23 capsular serotypes (**Table 2**).[23] The PPSV23 polysaccharide vaccine is indicated in select individuals more than 2 years of age, because it is not reliably immunogenic in children less than 2 years old. To bypass this problem, the pneumococcal conjugate vaccines were developed. The conjugate vaccines

Table 2
Comparison of serotypes contained in 13-valent pneumococcal conjugate and PPSV23 vaccines

Pneumococcal Vaccine	Serotypes Included
13-Valent pneumococcal conjugate vaccine (conjugated)	**1, 3, 4, 5, 6A, 6B, 7F, 9V, 14, 18C, 19A, 19F, 23F**
PPSV23 (polysaccharide)	**1,** 2, **3, 4, 5, 6B, 7F,** *8,* *9N,* **9V,** *10A,* *11A,* *12F,* **14,** *15B,* *17F,* **18C, 19A, 19F,** *20,* *22F,* **23F,** *33F*

Serotypes in bold are present in both.

generate a T-cell–dependent antibody response and are effective in children younger than 2 years of age.[23] The newer conjugated pneumococcal vaccine contains 13 serotypes.[34] The availability of different vaccines with different antigenic serotypes makes it difficult to standardize criteria for normal responses.

A working group report on diagnostic vaccination in PIDD recommends that a normal response to pneumococcal vaccines is a response to 50% or greater of serotypes for patients under 6 years of age, and a response to 70% or greater of serotypes for patients more than 6 years of age.[28] In support of these specified thresholds, the meta-analysis of pneumococcal responses in healthy individuals showed that the majority of patients could mount at least a 2-fold response to most serotypes.[30] Other studies report an adequate response as 1.3 μg/mL or greater for more than 50% of serotypes.[13,33]

Phenotypes of Specific Antibody Deficiency

Although questions remain regarding the definition of protective titers after vaccination to pneumococcal vaccines, guidelines from a working group report were developed using the best evidence available at the time to describe the diagnosis of SAD. Four clinical phenotypes were described, including mild, moderate, severe, and memory phenotype of deficient response, based on the response to PPSV23 (**Table 3**).[28] Patients with a

Table 3
Clinical phenotypes of SAD in response to PPSV23 polysaccharide vaccine

Phenotype[a]	Age >6 y	Age <6 y	Notes
Severe	<2 protective titers	<2 protective titers	Protective titers present are low
Moderate	<70% of serotypes protective	<50% of serotypes protective	Protective titers to >3 serotypes
Mild	Failure to generate protective titers to multiple serotypes or failure of a 2-fold increase in 70% of serotypes	Failure to generate protective titers to multiple serotypes or failure of a 2-fold increase in 50% of serotypes	2-fold increases assume a prevaccination titer of <4.4–10.3 μg/mL, depending on the pneumococcal serotype
Memory	Loss of response within 6 mo	Loss of response within 6 mo	Adequate initial response to >50% of serotypes in children <6 y of age and >70% in those >6 y of age

A protective response considered ≥1.3 μg/mL.
[a] All phenotypes assume a history of infection.

mild phenotype have multiple serotypes to which they did not generate protective titers, or were unable to increase titers by 2-fold. Patients with a moderate phenotype produce protective titers to more than 3 serotypes but to less than 50% of serotypes for those less than 6 years of age, or less than 70% of serotypes for those more than 6 years of age. A severe phenotype is described as producing protective titers against 2 or fewer serotypes, and those protective titers generated tend to be low. Patients with a memory phenotype of deficient pneumococcal response initially mount an adequate response to vaccination, but do not sustain the response beyond 6 months.

For the diagnosis of SAD, titers against pneumococcal vaccine serotypes must be measured before and after immunization (4 weeks after vaccination), and it is of greatest importance to consider whether the final antibody titer values are above the protective limits. Results should be interpreted in the context of vaccination history. The 2015 practice parameter from the American Academy of Allergy Asthma and Immunology (AAAAI), American College of Allergy, Asthma & Immunology, and Joint Council of Allergy, Asthma and Immunology recommend that, for patients who have previously received at least 1 dose of conjugate vaccine, normal antibody levels against serotypes in the conjugate vaccine do not exclude the diagnosis of SAD; thus, at least 6 serotypes should be tested that are present in PPSV23 only.[6] SAD may be a transient issue in some patients, especially in children under the age of 6, and may resolve over time; therefore, patients may need reassessments over time.[35,36]

Infections in Specific Antibody Deficiency

Recurrent infections with *S pneumoniae* is considered the main pathogen in SAD, causing infections such as otitis media, sinusitis, bronchitis, and pneumonia,[34] although documentation of upper and lower respiratory tract infections outside of pneumonia is poor. Sepsis, meningitis, and osteomyelitis may also occur, although less commonly. Infections with other common respiratory flora such as *H influenzae* and *Moraxella catarrhalis* are not well-documented in SAD, but are likely implicated given the nature of the antibody deficiency.[37]

Infections should be documented in as much detail as possible with appropriate culture and imaging data, and documentation of response to therapy. Other factors, including smoking, daycare attendance, and atopic disease, may affect the frequency and severity of respiratory infections and should be addressed.

The diagnosis of SAD should be considered in patients more than age 2 years with a history of documented recurrent respiratory tract infections, or serious infections with pneumococcus or other bacteria to which they have been vaccinated. Laboratory assessment includes quantitative Ig levels and vaccine titers.[6] If the IgG level is normal, but antibody titers to pneumococcal polysaccharides are absent or low, then unconjugated pneumococcal vaccination should be administered and postvaccine titers measured after approximately 4 weeks. If the 4 week postvaccination testing is abnormal, then intervention can be considered based on the severity of the hyporesponsiveness and clinical presentation. If the response is adequate, titers should be measured again 6 months after the vaccination in consideration of a possible memory phenotype of waning vaccination titers, or later if infections recur after initial improvement. If this assessment does not show substantive decreases in titer, then the diagnosis of SAD should not be considered further.

TREATMENT OF SPECIFIC ANTIBODY DEFICIENCY

A limited number of recommendations from consensus reports and expert opinion exist for the treatment of SAD (**Table 4**). Most cases of SAD present with a relatively

Table 4
Summary of therapeutic strategies for patients with SAD

Recommendation	2015 Practice Parameter for the Diagnosis and Management of Primary Immunodeficiency (AAAI, ACAAI, and JCAAI)[6]	Third National Immunoglobulin Database Report and Department of Health Recommendations (UK)[43,44]
General	Treatment decisions based on SAD phenotype	Not mentioned
Antibiotics	Intensified use of antibiotics may benefit	Antibiotics considered primary treatment
Immune globulin therapy	Select cases might benefit from a period of IgG replacement. For patients who have responded and stable, consider discontinuation after 1–2 y for 4–6 mo and reevaluation under the guidance of treating physician	Initiate treatment if approved by clinical immunologist and severe, persistent, opportunistic, or recurrent bacterial infections occur despite continuous oral antibiotic therapy for 3 mo, and there is documented failure of serum antibody response to unconjugated pneumococcal or other polysaccharide vaccine challenge
Vaccination	May benefit from additional immunization with conjugate pneumococcal vaccines. If they have not received the pneumococcal conjugate vaccine, vaccinate with conjugate vaccine having largest number of serotypes	Not mentioned

Abbreviations: ACAAI, American College of Allergy, Asthma & Immunology; JCAAI, Joint Council of Allergy, Asthma and Immunology.

mild clinical phenotype and the consensus is that these should be initially treated with antibiotic prophylaxis.

The 2015 practice parameter established by the American College of Allergy, Asthma & Immunology, the AAAAI, and the Joint Council of Allergy, Asthma and Immunology recommends that patients with SAD may benefit from additional immunization with conjugate pneumococcal vaccines.[6] If patients have not received the conjugate pneumococcal vaccine, immunization with the conjugate vaccine with the greatest number of serotypes available is recommended in all patients with recurrent infections. Even for patients who had received the conjugate vaccine earlier in childhood, repeating this vaccination might lead to the generation of antibody titers at a later point in life. The generation of titers from a conjugate vaccine, although not studied in a SAD population, should be measured and may provide therapeutic benefit. There are no standardized regimens for antibiotic prophylaxis or studies of efficacy. All practice is based on expert opinion, whether for antibiotic prophylaxis or repeat vaccination. Allergies are often present in patients with SAD and patients must be treated by standard interventions such as allergen avoidance, antihistamines, and topical steroids, along with treatments directed toward the defective antibody response. Gammaglobulin therapy may provide benefit to patients with SAD.[6,18,33,38] Regardless of phenotype, if infections continue despite appropriate management, immunoglobulin therapy may be indicated.[6,18,33,38] In children especially under the age of 6 with SAD who respond well to gammaglobulin therapy, reevaluation during a trial off gammaglobulin, after 1 to 2 years may help to determine whether therapy should be continued or if the immune system has overcome the SAD.[6,18,38]

Antibiotic Prophylaxis

There is little evidence to guide the use of antibiotic prophylaxis in patients with SAD. Current antibiotic prophylactic strategies are based on studies of immune competent patients with recurrent acute otitis media, chronic rhinosinusitis, cystic fibrosis, and bronchiectasis.[18] Although the majority of experts use antibiotic prophylaxis in practice,[39,40] studies are needed to determine the optimal dose, duration, and choice of antibiotic. The topic of prophylactic antibiotics in PIDD has recently been reviewed,[41] but SAD was not included in this discussion.

Antibiotic prophylaxis is often used to treat SAD. A survey of PIDD management of 405 allergists and immunologists in the United States was performed and the findings were reported separately for general and specialized immunologists (based on patients with PIDD comprising >10% of their clinical practice).[40] The majority reported using antibiotic prophylaxis in patients with SAD, with no significant difference in the percentage of general versus specialized immunologists using antibiotic prophylaxis. More than 50% of specialized immunologists considered antibiotic prophylaxis useful. Antibiotic prophylaxis should be considered the first-line therapy where pneumococcal conjugate vaccination fails to provide protection. There is no consensus protocol regarding the frequency and severity of infections that should motivate clinicians to begin antibiotic prophylaxis, so best clinical judgment and an individualized approach to the patient is necessary. (**Box 1**) Further discussions on the use of prophylactic antibiotics can be found in Refs.[39–42] Some patients may require year-round prophylaxis, whereas others do well with seasonal use of prophylactic antibiotics. Those who continue to have infections on antibiotic prophylaxis, or who cannot tolerate long-term antibiotics, should be considered as candidates for IgG supplementation.

IgG Replacement Therapy

Expert guidelines and opinions have recommended IgG therapy in patients with SAD.[6,18,33,38,43,44] Retrospective studies[14,45–47] also support IgG replacement therapy, although definitive data are lacking. The 2015 practice parameter for the diagnosis and management of primary immunodeficiency recommends that some patients with SAD might benefit from a period of IgG replacement therapy, based on immunologic and clinical severity, as well as unresponsiveness or adverse effects of other medical interventions.[6] Other parameters outlined by the UK Department of

---

Box 1
Antibiotic prophylaxis regimens

Azithromycin[a]
  Children – 5 mg/kg 3 times per week
  Adults – 250 or 500 mg 3 times per week

Sulfamethoxazole-trimethoprim
  Children - 5 mg/kg/d
  Adults - 160 mg/d

[a] Caution in adult patients using CYP3A inhibitors along with macrolides: cardiac side effects associated with prolonged repolarization resulting in QT prolongation may increase the risk of sudden death.

Health recommend that IgG therapy should be given only if antibiotic therapy is ineffective and impaired antibody production is demonstrated,[38,44] which is consistent with opinions from other experts.[18,33,38] Recommended doses of IgG for treatment of SAD are the same as those used to treat other PIDDs and are based on clinical outcome[38,44]; however, there are no evidence-based criteria to determine the optimal duration of IgG replacement therapy. The 2015 practice parameter for the diagnosis and management of primary immunodeficiency recommends that young patients who have stabilized after a period of IgG treatment, and are deemed at low risk for relapse, and should discontinue IgG treatment for a period of 4 to 6 months to reevaluate treatment.[6] Also, in some patients, IgA and IgM levels, total B-cell numbers, and proportions of memory B cells may also normalize over time and be used as a possible indicator of improvement in humoral immune function. Spontaneous resolution of humoral immunodeficiency is more common in children than in adults.

The effectiveness of IgG therapy in preventing infections in patients with SAD has been evaluated in retrospective studies,[45–47] but further studies are needed to optimize treatment strategies. The majority of immunologists in the US-based PIDD management survey reported using IgG therapy to treat at least some patients with SAD, and there was no significant difference in IgG use between specialized and general immunologists. Another survey was performed with experts from the AAAAI and ESID[39] that showed that approximately one-half of all immunologists recommended IgG therapy for at least 5% to 50% of patients with SAD and there was no significant difference between the percentages of specialized and general immunologists or in the percentages of experts from the AAAAI and ESID who prescribe IgG therapy. Although there is a lack of guidance regarding IgG use in patients with SAD, use is similar among immunologists. IgG therapy should be considered in those who have some combination of the following: severe or very frequent recurrent infections, poor response to pneumococcal polysaccharide vaccination, an inability to tolerate antibiotic prophylaxis owing to multiple hypersensitivity, severe side effects or complications such as *Clostridium difficile* colitis, or failure to respond to prophylactic antibiotics.

SUMMARY

Further studies are required to advance our understanding of SAD for improved diagnosis and management.[18,28] The prevalence of SAD in different age groups is unclear and further data, especially with regard to incidence in patients with specific types of infection, would aid diagnosis. SAD has often been considered an issue that may resolve with time, especially in children,[46] but in others it may evolve into more severe forms of humoral immunodeficiency such as CVID. Some evidence indicates that memory switched B-cell percentage is a good indicator of clinical complications associated with SAD[17]; however, it is not effective at classifying patients according to SAD or CVID diagnosis.

Further standardization of the diagnosis of SAD would also be extremely valuable and would facilitate accurate and early identification of patients, allowing for more effective therapeutic decisions. Variation in results from different laboratories also creates challenges for diagnosis based on the measurement of vaccine responses.[48] Decisions to treat SAD with prophylactic antibiotics and/or gammaglobulin replacement therapy are guided by clinical judgment, small studies, and recent consensus documents, which may evolve over time as more knowledge is gained.

DISCLOSURE

E.E. Perez: Consultancy and speaker bureau for CSL Behring, Takeda, Genentech; recent clinical trial PI or co-PI with Octapharma, Kedrion, Green Cross; M. Barrow: Physician advisory board and speaker bureau for CSL Behring, Takeda and Grifols; consulting medical director for the Immune Deficiency Foundation; Data Safety Monitoring Board – Prometic, Glenmark.

REFERENCES

1. Perez E, Bonilla FA, Orange JS, et al. Specific antibody deficiency: controversies in diagnosis and management. Front Immunol 2017;8:586 [Erratum in Front Immunol 2018;9:450].
2. Fried AJ, Bonilla FA. Pathogenesis, diagnosis, and management of primary antibody deficiencies and infections. Clin Microbiol Rev 2009;22(3):396–414.
3. Soresina A, Mahlaoui N, Wolska B, et al. ESID Registry Diagnosis Criteria. 2015. Available at: http://esid.org/Working-Parties/Registry/Diagnosis-criteria. Accessed December 14 2016.
4. Picard C, Al-Herz W, Bousfiha A, et al. Primary immunodeficiency diseases: an update on the classification from the International Union of Immunological Societies Expert Committee for Primary Immunodeficiency 2015. J Clin Immunol 2015;35(8):696–726.
5. Epstein MM, Gruskay F. Selective deficiency in pneumococcal antibody response in children with recurrent infections. Ann Allergy Asthma Immunol 1995;75(2): 125–31.
6. Bonilla FA, Khan DA, Ballas ZK, et al. Practice parameter for the diagnosis and management of primary immunodeficiency. J Allergy Clin Immunol 2015;136(5): 1186–205.
7. Leinonen M, Sakkinen A, Kalliokoski R, et al. Antibody response to 14-valent pneumococcal capsular polysaccharide vaccine in pre-school age children. Pediatr Infect Dis 1986;5(1):39–44.
8. Balloch A, Licciardi PV, Russell FM, et al. Infants aged 12 months can mount adequate serotype-specific IgG responses to pneumococcal polysaccharide vaccine. J Allergy Clin Immunol 2010;126(2):395–7.
9. Modell V, Knaus M, Modell F, et al. Global overview of primary immunodeficiencies: a report from Jeffrey Modell Centers worldwide focused on diagnosis, treatment, and discovery. Immunol Res 2014;60(1):132–44.
10. Hidalgo H, Moore C, Leiva LE, et al. Preimmunization and postimmunization pneumococcal antibody titers in children with recurrent infections. Ann Allergy Asthma Immunol 1996;76(4):341–6.
11. Sanders LA, Rijkers GT, Kuis W, et al. Defective antipneumococcal polysaccharide antibody response in children with recurrent respiratory tract infections. J Allergy Clin Immunol 1993;91(1 Pt 1):110–9.
12. Javier FC 3rd, Moore CM, Sorensen RU. Distribution of primary immunodeficiency diseases diagnosed in a pediatric tertiary hospital. Ann Allergy Asthma Immunol 2000;84(1):25–30.
13. Carr TF, Koterba AP, Chandra R, et al. Characterization of specific antibody deficiency in adults with medically refractory chronic rhinosinusitis. Am J Rhinol Allergy 2011;25(4):241–4.
14. Kashani S, Carr TF, Grammer LC, et al. Clinical characteristics of adults with chronic rhinosinusitis and specific antibody deficiency. J Allergy Clin Immunol Pract 2015;3(2):236–42.

15. Keswani A, Mehrotra N, Manzur A, et al. The clinical significance of specific anti-body deficiency (SAD) severity in chronic rhinosinusitis (CRS). J Allergy Clin Immunol 2014;133(2):AB236.

16. Ekdahl K, Braconier JH, Svanborg C. Immunoglobulin deficiencies and impaired immune response to polysaccharide antigens in adult patients with recurrent community-acquired pneumonia. Scand J Infect Dis 1997;29(4):401–7.

17. Alachkar H, Taubenheim N, Haeney MR, et al. Memory switched B cell percent-age and not serum immunoglobulin concentration is associated with clinical complications in children and adults with specific antibody deficiency and common variable immunodeficiency. Clin Immunol 2006;120(3):310–8.

18. Wall LA, Dimitriades VR, Sorensen RU. Specific antibody deficiencies. Immunol Allergy Clin North Am 2015;35(4):659–70.

19. Hanson EP, Monaco-Shawver L, Solt LA, et al. Hypomorphic nuclear factor-kappaB essential modulator mutation database and reconstitution system identifies phenotypic and immunologic diversity. J Allergy Clin Immunol 2008; 122(6):1169–77.

20. Bonilla FA, Barlan I, Chapel H, et al. International Consensus Document (ICON): common variable immunodeficiency disorders. J Allergy Clin Immunol Pract 2016;4(1):38–59.

21. Quezada A, Norambuena X, Inostroza J, et al. Specific antibody deficiency with normal immunoglobulin concentration in children with recurrent respiratory infections. Allergol Immunopathol (Madr) 2015;43(3):292–7.

22. US Department of Health and Human Services; Centres for Disease Control and Prevention. Pneumococcal vaccine timing for adults. 2015. Available at: https://www.cdc.gov/vaccines/vpd/pneumo/downloads/pneumo-vaccine-timing.pdf. Accessed December 19, 2016.

23. Daniels CC, Rogers PD, Shelton CM. A review of pneumococcal vaccines: current polysaccharide vaccine recommendations and future protein antigens. J Pediatr Pharmacol Ther 2016;21(1):27–35.

24. Elberse KE, Tcherniaeva I, Berbers GA, et al. Optimization and application of a multiplex bead-based assay to quantify serotype-specific IgG against Streptococcus pneumoniae polysaccharides: response to the booster vaccine after immunization with the pneumococcal 7-valent conjugate vaccine. Clin Vaccin Immunol 2010;17(4):674–82.

25. Klein DL, Martinez JE, Hickey MH, et al. Development and characterization of a multiplex bead-based immunoassay to quantify pneumococcal capsular polysaccharide-specific antibodies. Clin Vaccin Immunol 2012;19(8):1276–82.

26. Jeurissen A, Moens L, Raes M, et al. Laboratory diagnosis of specific antibody deficiency to pneumococcal capsular polysaccharide antigens. Clin Chem 2007;53(3):505–10.

27. Koskela M, Leinonen M. Comparison of ELISA and RIA for measurement of pneumococcal antibodies before and after vaccination with 14-valent pneumococcal capsular polysaccharide vaccine. J Clin Pathol 1981;34(1):93–8.

28. Orange JS, Ballow M, Stiehm ER, et al. Use and interpretation of diagnostic vaccination in primary immunodeficiency: a working group report of the Basic and Clinical Immunology Interest Section of the American Academy of Allergy, Asthma & Immunology. J Allergy Clin Immunol 2012;130(3 Suppl):S1–24.

29. Sorensen RU, Leiva LE, Javier FC 3rd, et al. Influence of age on the response to Streptococcus pneumoniae vaccine in patients with recurrent infections and normal immunoglobulin concentrations. J Allergy Clin Immunol 1998;102(2): 215–21.

30. Go ES, Ballas ZK. Anti-pneumococcal antibody response in normal subjects: a meta-analysis. J Allergy Clin Immunol 1996;98(1):205–15.

31. World Health Organization. Weekly epidemiological record. 2012;87:129–44. Available at: https://www.who.int/wer/en/.

32. Bonilla FA, Bernstein IL, Khan DA, et al. Practice parameter for the diagnosis and management of primary immunodeficiency. Ann Allergy Asthma Immunol 2005; 94(5 Suppl 1):S1–63.

33. Ocampo CJ, Peters AT. Antibody deficiency in chronic rhinosinusitis: epidemiology and burden of illness. Am J Rhinol Allergy 2013;27(1):34–8.

34. Sorensen RW, Harvey T, Leiva LE. Selective antibody deficiency with normal immunoglobulins. In: Metodiev K, editor. Immunodeficiency. Rijeka (Croatia): InTech; 2012. p. 191–205.

35. Bonilla FA, Notarangelo LD. Primary immunodeficiency diseases. In: Orkin SH, Nathan DG, Ginsburg D, et al, editors. Nathan and Oski's hematology and oncology of infancy and childhood. 8th edition. Philadelphia: Elsevier Saunders; 2015. p. 886–922.

36. Koskela M, Leinonen M, Haiva VM, et al. First and second dose antibody responses to pneumococcal polysaccharide vaccine in infants. Pediatr Infect Dis 1986;5(1):45–50.

37. Kainulainen L, Nikoskelainen J, Vuorinen T, et al. Viruses and bacteria in bronchial samples from patients with primary hypogammaglobulinemia. Am J Respir Crit Care Med 1999;159(4 Pt 1):1199–204.

38. Garcia-Lloret M, McGhee S, Chatila TA. Immunoglobulin replacement therapy in children. Immunol Allergy Clin North Am 2008;28(4):833–49.

39. Hernandez-Trujillo HS, Chapel H, Lo Re V 3rd, et al. Comparison of American and European practices in the management of patients with primary immunodeficiencies. Clin Exp Immunol 2012;169(1):57–69.

40. Yong PL, Boyle J, Ballow M, et al. Use of intravenous immunoglobulin and adjunctive therapies in the treatment of primary immunodeficiencies: a working group report of and study by the Primary Immunodeficiency Committee of the American Academy of Allergy Asthma and Immunology. Clin Immunol 2010;135(2):255–63.

41. Kuruvilla M, de la Morena MT. Antibiotic prophylaxis in primary immune deficiency disorders. J Allergy Clin Immunol Pract 2013;1(6):573–82.

42. Ballow M, Paris K, de la Morena M. Should antibiotic prophylaxis be routinely used in patients with antibody mediated primary immunodeficiency? J Allergy Clin Immunol Pract 2018;6:421–6.

43. Third National Immunoglobulin Database Report (2012) National Health Service, UK. 2013. Available at: http://www.ivig.nhs.uk/documents/Third_National_Immunoglobulin_Database_Report_2011_2012.pdf. Accessed December 14, 2016.

44. Guidelines for Immunoglobulin Use. Department of Health, UK. 2nd edition. 2011. Available at: http://www.ivig.nhs.uk/documents/dh_129666.pdf. Accessed December 14, 2016.

45. Cheng YK, Decker PA, O'Byrne MM, et al. Clinical and laboratory characteristics of 75 patients with specific polysaccharide antibody deficiency syndrome. Ann Allergy Asthma Immunol 2006;97(3):306–11.

46. Ruuskanen O, Nurkka A, Helminen M, et al. Specific antibody deficiency in children with recurrent respiratory infections: a controlled study with follow-up. Clin Exp Immunol 2013;172(2):238–44.

47. Schwartz HJ, Hostoffer RW, McFadden ER Jr, et al. The response to intravenous immunoglobulin replacement therapy in patients with asthma with specific antibody deficiency. Allergy Asthma Proc 2006;27(1):53–8.
48. Daly TM, Pickering JW, Zhang X, et al. Multilaboratory assessment of threshold versus fold-change algorithms for minimizing analytical variability in multiplexed pneumococcal IgG measurements. Clin Vaccin Immunol 2014;21(7):982–8.

Precision Therapy for the Treatment of Primary Immunodysregulatory Diseases

Deepak Chellapandian, MD, MBBS[a], Maria Chitty-Lopez, MD[b], Jennifer W. Leiding, MD[b],*

KEYWORDS

- Biologic modifiers • Precision therapy • Hemophagocytic lymphohistiocytosis
- Signal transducer and activator of transcription 1 gain of function
- Signal transducer and activator of transcription 3 gain of function
- Cytotoxic T-lymphocyte antigen 4
- Lipopolysaccharide-responsive beige-like anchor

KEY POINTS

- Primary immunodysregulatory disorders are an expanding group of molecularly defined primary immunodeficiency diseases in which autoimmunity and hyperinflammation are hallmarks.
- Cytotoxic T-lymphocyte antigen 4 (CTLA4)-Ig fusion proteins serve as a functional replacement of CTLA-4, successfully treating patients with CTLA4 haploinsufficiency and LRBA deficiency.
- Leniolisib (CDZ173), a potent inhibitor of the p110δ subunit of PI3Kδ, has successfully treated lymphoproliferation in patients with activated PI3K deficiency syndrome.
- Jakinibs inhibit Janus kinase– signal transducer and activator of transcription (STAT) activation, successfully improving disease-related manifestations in patients with STAT1 gain of function (GOF) and STAT3-GOF.
- Precision therapy provides targeted therapeutic medications that alter the aberrant immune response, leading to improvement or resolution of disease-related manifestations.

INTRODUCTION

Precision therapy is a concept in which medical treatment is tailored to the patient's individual needs based on individual characteristics and mechanism of disease. Primary immunodysregulatory disorders (PIRDs) are an expanding group of primary

[a] Blood and Marrow Transplant Program, Johns Hopkins University School of Medicine, Johns Hopkins All Children's Hospital, Research and Education Building, 600 5th Street South, 4th Floor, St Petersburg, FL 33701, USA; [b] Division of Allergy and Immunology, Department of Pediatrics, University of South Florida, Children's Research Institute, 601 – 4th Street South, CRI 4008, St Petersburg, FL 33701, USA
* Corresponding author.
E-mail address: jleiding@usf.edu

Immunol Allergy Clin N Am 40 (2020) 511–526
https://doi.org/10.1016/j.iac.2020.04.001
0889-8561/20/© 2020 Elsevier Inc. All rights reserved.

immunodeficiency diseases that are characterized by early onset autoimmunity and autoinflammation. In many cases of PIRDs, alteration of the aberrant immune response by application of precise therapeutic medications has shown clinical efficacy in resolving disease-related manifestations. This article reviews targeted precision-based therapy for the treatment of PIRDs (**Table 1**).

CYTOTOXIC T LYMPHOCYTE ANTIGEN-4 HAPLOINSUFFICIENCY

Cytotoxic T-lymphocyte antigen 4 (CTLA-4) is a key negative immune regulator crucial for the function of regulatory T (Treg) cells that are responsible for maintaining self-tolerance and immune homeostasis.[1] CTLA4 competes with the costimulatory receptor CD28 for its ligands CD80 and CD86 on antigen-presenting cells (APCs). Upon binding, CTLA4 reduces the expression of CD28, resulting in reduction of APC-mediated activation of T cells, thereby downregulating the immune response.

CTLA4 haploinsufficiency is caused by heterozygous germline mutations in *CTLA4*, which results in a disease of immune dysregulation and susceptibility to infections.

Table 1
Targeted therapies used in the treatment of PIDD

Drug	Molecular Target	Molecular Structure	Use in Immunodeficiency Diseases
Sirolimus	mTOR	Macrolide compound	NLCR4-GOF CTLA-4 haploinsufficiency APDS
Abatacept	B7-1 (CD80), B7-2 (CD86)	CTLA-4 IgG fusion protein	CTLA-4 haploinsufficiency LRBA deficiency
Belatacept	B7-1 (CD80), B7-2 (CD86)	CTLA-4 IgG fusion protein	CTLA-4 haploinsufficiency
Anakinra	IL-1R	Recombinant human IL-1R antagonist	Cryopyrin associated periodic fever syndromes
Canakinumab	IL-1β	Antihuman IL-1 IgG1 monoclonal antibody	DIRA
Rilonacept	IL-1β	IgG1 linked to IL-1R and IL-1R accessory protein	DIRA
Tocilizumab	IL-6R	IgG1κ recombinant humanized monoclonal antibody	STAT3-GOF
Ruxolitinib	JAK1 and JAK 2	Small molecule inhibitor	STAT3-GOF STAT1-GOF
Tofacitinib	JAK 1 and JAK3	Small molecule inhibitor	STAT3-GOF STAT1-GOF
Baricitinib	JAK1 and JAK 2	Small molecule inhibitor	STAT1-GOF
Tadekinig-alfa	IL-18 binding protein	Recombinant IL-18 binding protein	NLCR4-GOF
Leniolisib	PI3Kδ	Small molecule inhibitor	APDS

Kuehn and colleagues[2] originally described 7 patients from 4 families with CTLA-4 haploinsufficiency. Most patients presented with clinical and laboratory findings consistent with common variable immunodeficiency (CVID), manifesting with hypogammaglobulinemia, autoimmune cytopenias (AIC), and lymphocytic infiltration of nonlymphoid organs. Patients also exhibited progressive reduction of B cells with an increased proportion of autoreactive CD21[low] B cells. CTLA-4 haploinsufficiency is characterized by incomplete penetrance and variable expressivity.[3] More recently, Schwab and colleagues[4] described the largest cohort of 133 subjects with CTLA-4 haploinsufficiency with a penetrance of 60% to 70%. The median age of onset was 11 years, and patients manifested with hypogammaglobulinemia, lymphoproliferation, autoimmune multilineage cell cytopenias, and lymphoid malignancies. Most patients had pulmonary and gastrointestinal (GI) disease. Respiratory tract manifestations included recurrent lower and upper respiratory tract infections, granulomatous lymphocytic interstitial lung disease, bronchiectasis, and idiopathic lung fibrosis. GI manifestations included severe enteropathy and Crohn-like disease. AICs were often severe and life-threatening. The immune phenotype is variable, but most often includes hypogammaglobulinemia, impaired response to immunizations, low numbers of CD4 T cells, and defective B cell maturation.[2,4]

Fusion proteins like abatacept and belatacept and mechanistic target of rapamycin (mTOR) inhibitors have shown to be an effective targeted treatment to control immune dysregulation in CTLA4 deficient patients (see **Table 1**).[5] Abatacept and belatacept are fusion proteins that contain an extracellular domain of CTLA-4 and the Fc portion of human immunoglobulin G (IgG)1 (CTLA-4-Fc-IgG1) and serve as a replacement for functional loss of CTLA4. Lee and colleagues[6] reported the effectiveness of abatacept in an adolescent girl with a functional mutation in CTLA4 who had chronic diarrhea, autoimmune enteropathy, megaloblastic anemia, and autoimmune hepatitis. Treatment with abatacept resulted in improvement of diarrhea and resolution of Coombs-positive hemolytic anemia and led to discontinuation of other immunosuppressive agents. Abatacept or belatacept was used to treat 11 additional patients reported in the Schwab and colleagues cohort. Patients were reported to have resolution of lymphoproliferation in the lung with improvement in respiratory symptoms, reduced lymph node size, and reduced diarrhea with notable weight gain. Abatacept was also successfully used to treat steroid-refractory intracerebral T cell-mediated inflammation in a 20-year-old man with CTLA4 deficiency who presented with CVID-like disease.[7]

Sirolimus (mTOR inhibitor) has been used to inhibit the CD28 signaling pathway, thereby decreasing T cell hyperactivity and immune dysregulation and has been used with success in treatment of autoimmune lymphoproliferative disease (ALPS) (see **Table 1**).[8] In CTLA-4 deficiency, 13 patients who were treated with sirolimus[4] had improvement of AIC, regression of lymphadenopathy and splenomegaly, and decreased consumption of immunoglobulin. Vedolizumab, a humanized monoclonal antibody that targets T cells expressing the gut homing receptor, $\alpha 4\beta 7$ integrin, has also been successfully used in treating refractory autoimmune enterocolitis in a patient with CTLA4 deficiency; however, vedolizumab did not reverse the hypogammaglobulinemia and pure red cell aplasia that were also present in the same patient.[9]

The use of abatacept and belatacept in CTLA4 deficiency appears to be a promising first-line therapy to control manifestations of immune dysregulation; however, the lifelong use of this therapy is limited by increased susceptibility to infections and possible evolution of malignancies.[10] For these reasons, hematopoietic cell transplantation (HCT) should be carefully considered as a possible definitive therapy in patients with CTLA4 deficiency. Slatter and colleagues[11] described HCT in 8 patients with

CTLA4 deficiency. The diagnosis was made retrospectively in 7 of 8 patients who underwent HCT for life-threatening treatment-refractory immune dysregulation. All received 10/10 HLA-matched unrelated donors following reduced-intensity conditioning regimens. Six of the 8 patients are alive and well, with donor chimerism ranging 85% to 100%. Results from this study are encouraging, despite the small cohort of patients, supporting the idea that HCT may represent an optimal therapy in patients with a severe disease phenotype.

LIPOPOLYSACCHARIDE-RESPONSIVE BEIGE-LIKE ANCHOR DEFICIENCY

Lipopolysaccharide-responsive beige-like anchor (LRBA) deficiency leads to an autosomal-recessive form of combined immunodeficiency, caused by biallelic mutations in *LRBA* gene.[12,13] LRBA is a ubiquitously expressed cytosolic protein that regulates the traffic of intracellular vesicles and is involved in the endocytosis of ligand-activated receptors. CTLA-4 undergoes endocytosis within T cells, where it is either recycled back to the plasma membrane or degraded within lysosomes. LRBA normally prevents CTLA-4 from lysosomal degradation by bringing it back to the cell surface. Absence of LRBA leads to decreased CTLA4 expression, thereby resulting in defective Treg cell function, causing immune dysregulation and autoimmunity.[14]

LRBA deficiency was originally reported in 2012 in 4 consanguineous families who presented with early onset antibody deficiency and autoimmunity.[15] The immunologic phenotype is characterized by hypogammaglobulinemia with normal B cell quantities but low switched memory B cells. Patients with LRBA deficiency and CTLA-4 deficiency share phenotypic similarities. With LRBA deficiency, patients usually present early in life with infections, autoimmunity, and hypogammaglobulinemia. Since the original description, the clinical phenotype of this disease has expanded to include immunodysregulation-polyendocrinopathy-enteropathy-X-linked (IPEX) disease-like symptoms, AICs, lymphocytic interstitial pneumonia, and early onset diabetes.[16,17] Autoimmune hepatitis, myasthenia gravis, uveitis, alopecia, polyarthritis, and gastric adenocarcinoma have also been reported.[13,18,19] Central nervous system (CNS) manifestations have been rarely reported but have included demyelination, brain atrophy, and granulomas.[16]

The functional interplay of LRBA and CTLA4 in T cell homeostasis has provided the rationale to treat both conditions using abatacept (see **Table 1**). Use of this treatment in 3 LRBA-deficient patients led to reversal of lymphocytic interstitial lung disease and cytopenias, but not enteropathy that required additional treatment with sirolimus and other immunosuppressant drugs.[14] Symptoms of lymphoproliferation, enteropathy, and autoimmune cytopenias responded the most to treatment with abatacept in a large Turkish cohort.[20,21] Dosing frequency of abatacept is also important for symptom resolution. More frequent weekly dosing leads to higher disease manifestation resolution.[20] Treatment with abatacept results in improvement in immunologic phenotype as shown by increasing naive effector T-cell ratios, improved functional antibody responses to polysaccharide vaccines, and reduced circulating T follicular helper (cT$_{FH}$) cell quantities. Further cT$_{FH}$ quantities correlate with disease activity.[14,20] In vitro studies have demonstrated that chloroquine, an inhibitor of lysosomal degradation, may also reverse CTLA4 expression loss, suggesting its potential role as an immunomodulatory drug in the treatment of this disease.[14,20,21]

HCT is the only potentially curative treatment, as with CTLA-4 deficiency; however, few patients with LRBA deficiency have been transplanted to date.[16,22,23] Tesch and colleagues[23] recently described the largest cohort of 76 patients with LRBA deficiency, 24 of whom underwent HCT. The median time between onset of disease and transplantation was 7.4 years (range 0.4–15.8 years). The disease burden and treatment response were assessed using a specialized scoring system. A favorable degree of disease remission was observed in the HCT cohort (70.6%) compared with patients who were treated on immunosuppressive therapy alone (11.6%). Lung involvement and AICs significantly correlated with a fatal disease outcome in this disease. The HCT outcomes were significantly better in patients with low disease score, underscoring the importance of early and careful consideration of HCT before the onset of organ-specific lymphoproliferation, particularly of the lung.

ACTIVATED PI3K DEFICIENCY SYNDROME

Activated P13K deficiency syndrome (APDS) is a combined immunodeficiency syndrome associated with multiple noninfectious complications such as nonmalignant lymphoproliferation (lymphadenopathy, hepatosplenomegaly, nodular mucosal lymphoid hyperplasia), increased risk for lymphoma and other malignancies, developmental delay, and autoimmune and inflammatory diseases.[24] Phosphoinositide-3-kinase δ (PI3Kδ) is a class IA lipid kinase that phosphorylates phosphatidylinositol-4,5-bisphosphate (PIP2) to produce phosphatidylinositol-3,4,5-trisphosphate (PIP3). PI3Kδ has an important role in downstream signaling of the T cell and B cell antigen receptor, Toll-like receptor, and intracellular signaling of myeloid cells.[25]

APDS is caused by autosomal-dominant (AD) gain-of-function (GOF) mutations in genes encoding p110δ (*PIK3CD*) catalytic subunit or p85 (*PIK3R1*) regulatory subunit of PI3Kδ.[25,26] APDS-1, because of a GOF mutation in *PIK3CD*, was initially described in 2013 by Angulo and colleagues,[25] who described a cohort of 17 patients with frequent respiratory infections, lymphopenia, increased circulating transitional B cells, elevated IgM, and decreased IgG.

Further immune characterization was shown by Lucas and colleagues,[26] who presented a cohort of 14 patients who had increased susceptibility to respiratory tract infections, severe disseminated viral infections, especially to Epstein-Barr virus (EBV) and cytomegalovirus (CMV), and a tendency to develop nonmalignant lymphoproliferation. In regard to their T cell compartment, these patients showed depletion of the naïve and central T cell memory branch with expansion of senescent effector T cells. In vitro T cell analysis revealed overactivation of mTOR increased glucose uptake and terminal effector differentiation. APDS-2, caused by a GOF mutation in *PIK3R1*, was subsequently described with similar clinical characteristics of recurrent respiratory tract infections, lymphoproliferation, and antibody deficiency.[27]

Conventional treatment of APDS includes antibiotic prophylaxis and immunoglobulin replacement therapy. Immunoglobulin dosing is recommended at 0.4 g/kg/mo in antibody-deficient patients without bronchiectasis and at a higher dose of 0.6 g/kg/mo in patients with bronchiectasis.[28]

Aiming to tackle associated nonmalignant lymphoproliferation, anti-CD20 monoclonal antibody (rituximab) and mTOR inhibitors (eg, rapamycin) have been employed with good response of reduction in splenomegaly and lymphadenopathy in APDS individuals.[26,29] Maccari and colleagues[29] showed favorable outcomes with use of rapamycin in APDS with reduction in non-neoplastic lymphoproliferative disease; 32% (8 of 25 cases) had complete response and 44% (11 of 25 cases) had partial response. Unfortunately treatment with mTOR inhibitors was not as beneficial in managing APDS-related cytopenias or APDS-related GI disease.

The understanding of APDS mechanism of disease presented the opportunity of targeted therapy with the use of selective PI3Kδ inhibitors: idelalisib, leniolisib, and nemiralisib.[28,30] PI3Kδ inhibitors were developed for oncologic therapy and inflammatory disease treatment including rheumatoid arthritis, asthma, and chronic obstructive pulmonary disease (COPD).[31–33] Leniolisib (CDZ173) is a potent oral inhibitor of the p110δ subunit of PI3Kδ, currently in clinical trials for the treatment of APDS (NCT02435173) (see **Table 1**). Rao and colleagues[34] recently reported the outcome of 6 APDS patients receiving CDZ173 in an open-label 12 week trial. Results showed a dose-dependent ex vivo reduction in PI3K/AKT pathway activity and a positive response in treatment of immune dysregulation. Treatment with CDZ173 led to normalization of the immune phenotype: normal transitional and naive B cell quantities, reduction in PD-1+CD4+ and senescent CD57+CD4- T-cells, decrease in previously elevated IgM, and decrease in inflammatory markers. By the trial's end, patients showed a significant reduction in lymph node sizes and spleen volume. An increase in patient wellbeing, decrease in patient fatigue, and less disease activity were reported by patients and physicians, respectively. Five out of 6 patients are now enrolled in a follow-up open-label long-term extension study with leniolisib. During the first 9 months of leniolisib use, there was no report of significant adverse effects.[34]

Nemiralisib, an inhaled PI3Kδ inhibitor, is currently being investigated as an anti-inflammatory treatment of chronic obstructive pulmonary disease (COPD) (NCT02593539). In APDS, It is proposed to be a candidate for directed therapy to be used in patients with lymphoproliferation and respiratory disease with a goal to reduce progression of bronchiectasis.[28,30,32] Idelalisib, an orally active selective PI3Kδ inhibitor, is currently approved for treatment of chronic lymphocytic leukemia and non-Hodgkin lymphoma. It has an adverse effect profile that includes pneumonitis, elevated transaminases, and colitis. Given safety concerns, idelalisib may only be appropriate if administered at lower doses or topically.[26,35]

HCT has also been explored as a treatment option of APDS. Nademi and colleagues[36] reported outcomes of HCT in 11 patients with APDS and severe combined immune deficiency. Age of the recipients ranged from 5 to 23 years. A total of 81% (9/11) of patients survived, and 8 had full immune reconstitution with discontinuation of immunoglobulin replacement therapy.

SIGNAL TRANSDUCTION AND ACTIVATOR OF TRANSCRIPTION 1 AND 3 – GAIN OF FUNCTION

The signal transducer and activator of transcription (STAT) family is composed of several transcription factors involved in activation of Janus kinase (JAK) signaling (**Fig. 1**).

Cellular signaling begins with cytokine and/or growth factor association to a transmembrane receptor, which stimulates the activation of receptor-bound JAKs. Cytosolic STATs are then tyrosine-phosphorylated by activated JAKs, prompting STAT dimerization, and such conformational change allows STAT nuclear translocation. Once in the nucleus, STATs can attach to gene-activating transcription promoters, subsequently modifying the immune response.

A total of 4 JAKs (JAK1, JAK2, JAK3, TYK2) and 7 STATs (STAT1, STAT2, STAT3, STAT4, STAT5a, STAT5b, STAT6) are used by more than 50 cytokines and growth factors in mammals.[37] Furthermore, the understanding of the JAK/STAT pathway's biological relevance has been determined by the study of germline mutations in the genes encoding 2 of the 4 human *JAKs* (*JAK3 and TYK2*) and 3 of the 6 human STATs (*STAT1, STAT3, and STAT5B*).[38] *STAT1* and *STAT3* defects can be caused by either loss-of function (LOF) or GOF mutations.[38] *STAT5B* has been mainly described in the context of deficiency.[39]

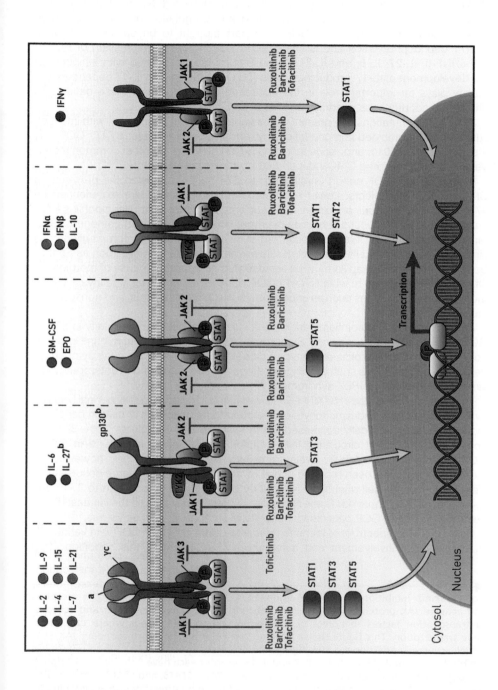

STAT 1 gain of function

STAT1 is specifically activated by type I and II interferons (IFN), interleukin (IL) 6, γ chain cytokines, IL-10, and IL-23, promoting an upregulation of IFN-γ-dependent genes. The overdrive in *STAT1* GOF is in part thought to be caused by lack of *STAT1* dephosphorylation and is characterized by increased expression of PDL-1, INF-α/INF-β, IL-27, IL-6, and IL-21. These factors are associated with inhibition of the development of IL-17-producing T cells (TH17). Deficiency in IL-17 dependent immunity plays an important role in the increased susceptibility of these patients to chronic mucocutaneous candidiasis (CMC).[40–42]

STAT1 GOF mutations can present with a variable clinical phenotype, with infection susceptibility, combined immunodeficiency, and IPEX-like disease. *STAT1* GOF was first described in 2011, and, since then, has been known as the most common monogenic cause of inherited CMC independent of demographic factors.[43,44]

A large *STAT1* GOF cohort enrolling up to 274 patients showed the presence of CMC in 98% of subjects. Lower respiratory tract infections were experienced by 47% with *Streptococcus pneumoniae, Pseudomonas aeruginosa, Haemophilus influenzae*, and *Staphylococcus aureus* as the most commonly identified pathogens. Systemic or recurrent viral infections occurred in 38% of cases, most commonly herpes simplex virus and varicella-zoster virus. However, other DNA viruses such as Epstein Barr virus and human papilloma virus represented an important cause of morbidity.[43] Other severe infections to which *STAT1* GOF patients are prone include invasive dysmorphic fungal infections such as coccidiomycosis, histoplasmosis, and non tuberculous mycobacteria.[40,45]

Autoimmunity and autoinflammation are a substantial cause of morbidity in *STAT1* GOF patients affecting nearly half. Symptoms often manifest as autoimmune endocrinopathies (eg, hypothyroidism and type I diabetes mellitus), autoimmune cytopenias, dermatologic conditions such as vitiligo or alopecia, and autoimmune enteropathy in a similar presentation as IPEX syndrome.[43,46]

The immune phenotype of *STAT1* GOF is variable but includes mostly normal lymphocyte subpopulations and lymphocyte proliferation to mitogens. Th17 cells in peripheral blood are characteristically decreased in the vast majority of patients (75%–82%). In conjunction, increased circulating INF-γ CD4+ T cells have been found in *STAT1* GOF patients. Immunoglobulin levels are mostly within normal ranges; however, low memory B cells have been reported in half of the patients[43,44] in a large cohort study. Despite normal NK cell quantities, NK cell cytolytic activity in response to IL-15 and IL-2 is significantly impaired. These findings can presumably explain the increased susceptibility of *STAT1* GOF patients to intracellular pathogens such as viruses.[47]

Given the wide spectrum of immune deficiency seen in *STAT1* GOF with variable T, B, and NK cell involvement and autoimmunity, treatment of this condition often

---

Fig. 1. Jakinib inhibition of JAK-STAT signaling. Cytokines bind their respective receptors and activate JAK proteins, which, in turn, phosphorylate signal transducer and activator of transcription factors to homo- or heterodimerize to the nucleus where they direct gene transcription. This figure shows selected cytokines and the corresponding JAK-STAT signal activated. Additionally, this figure shows where specific JAK inhibitors (jakinibs) inhibit the activated JAK protein. [a] IL-2 and IL-15 receptor each have 3 chains. [b] IL-27 signals through the gp130 receptor chain and can activate STAT1, STAT3, and STAT5. (*From* Leiding JW, Forbes LR. Mechanism-based precision therapy for the treatment of primary immunodeficiency and primary immunodysregulatory diseases. J Allergy Clin Immunol Pract 2019;7(3):765; with permission.)

requires a multidisciplinary approach. Infection prophylaxis remains a strong recommendation in the management of these patients. Long-term antifungal use is indicated as first-line treatment in the management of CMC. Antibiotic prophylaxis and immunoglobulin replacement therapy are employed in patients with recurrent respiratory tract infection despite lack of antibody deficiency.[43]

HCT, has been curative in patient with *STAT1* GOF. However, available data show only 40% of success when HCT was performed as a lifesaving treatment aiming to reverse severe infections, hemophagocytic lymphohistiocytosis (HLH), or autoimmunity with a high rate of secondary graft loss. HLH was observed to be a poor predictor of survival after HCT. More studies are needed to assess HCT outcomes in *STAT 1* GOF, especially when performed as an elective treatment, as disease-related morbidity seems to impact the overall survival.[48]

Mechanism-based precision therapies in *STAT1* GOF have become recently available and have shown promising results, especially addressing autoinflammatory manifestations of *STAT1* GOF. Tofacinitib, ruxolotinib, and baricitinib are inhibitors of JAK-STAT activation, also denominated jakinibs (see **Table 1**).[49,50]

A recent cohort of 11 patients with *STAT1* GOF with multiple autoimmune complications treated with ruxolitinib showed favorable clinical outcomes. CMC was present in 5 patients and disseminated coccidiomycosis in 1 patient. Six patients had autoimmune cytopenias or autoimmune hepatitis, and five had autoimmune enteropathy with associated growth failure. Most patients (10/11) receiving ruxolotinib in this cohort had substantial improvement in their immune dysregulatory *STAT1* GOF manifestations and CMC.[49] In addition to substantial improvement or resolution of immunodysregulatory symptoms, in vivo treatment with ruxolitinib has led to reduced hyperresponsiveness to type I and II interferons, normalization of Th1 and follicular T helper cell responses, improvement of Th17 differentiation,[51] improvement in NK cell perforin expression, NK cell cytolytic function, and JAK-STAT1 inhibition[49] in vitro. Barcitinib and tofacitinib have shown similar efficacy.[50]

Precautions with the use of jakinibs include liver profile monitoring, thrombocytopenia surveillance, systemic viral infection monitoring, and antiviral prophylaxis in order to mitigate the risk of herpes virus infections.[49]

STAT3 GAIN OF FUNCTION

STAT3 modulates the intracellular signaling of several cytokines (IFNs, IL-2, IL-6, IL-7, IL-10, IL-12, IL-15, IL-21, IL-23, and IL-27) and growth factors. STAT3 activation favors Th17cell response by increasing the expression of orphan nuclear receptors (RORγ/RORα), which are important transcription factors for Th17 cell activation and expansion. Activation of STAT3 also leads to restriction of regulatory T cell development.[52–54]

GOF germline mutations in *STAT3* cause an immunodeficiency characterized by immune dysregulation that is reminiscent of STAT5b-deficiency, ALPS, and IPEX-syndrome. The autoimmunity is attributed to *STAT3* hyperactivity causing Treg dysfunction.[55]

First described in 2014, Flanagan and colleagues[53] identified *STAT3* GOF mutations for the first time in 5 patients presenting with early onset (<5 years of age) diabetes. The disease phenotype was characterized further by 2 independent groups. Disease manifestations included early onset autoimmune disease, nonmalignant lymphoproliferation, and postnatal growth failure.[56,57] AICs, early onset diabetes, and autoimmune enteropathy were the most common autoimmune manifestations. Immune parameters are variable but include expanded populations of double-negative T cells (CD4-CD8-), hypogammaglobulinemia, lymphopenia, decrease in CD19+CD27+IgD-IgM-switched memory B cells, and reduced Treg cell populations.[56–58]

Added to their underlying immune dysfunction, these patients are usually exposed chronically to immunosuppressant drugs aiming to control their autoimmunity, all of which place them at an elevated risk for serious infections such as nontuberculous mycobacterium and systemic viral, opportunistic, and fungal infections.[50]

Given the dominant feature of immune dysregulation, and the fact that nonspecific immunosuppressive agents fail to control the disease,[49,53,56–58] precision-based therapy was considered soon after understanding the nature of the hyperactivity of STAT3 in patients with GOF germline mutations.[49]

In the Milner and colleagues[57] cohort a 10-year-old boy with autoimmune hemolytic anemia, polyarthritis, scleroderma, and autoimmune hepatitis was treated with tocilizumab, a humanized monoclonal antibody that targets IL-6 receptor. He displayed a dramatic improvement of his long-standing polyarthritis and scleroderma skin features over the first year of treatment. With the success of this 1 patient and the premise that IL-6 is increased in patients with STAT3-GOF, tocilzumab has been used as therapy in several additional patients. Treatment with tocilizumab was successful in stabilizing autoimmune hepatitis, interstitial lung disease, enteropathy, and lymphoproliferation. In addition to tocilizumab, and often used concurrently, treatment with jakinibs has been successful at reversing and/or controlling immunodysregulatory features.[49]

HCT in STAT3 GOF has been reported in only 5 subjects. One had full immune reconstitution with remission of autoimmunity. Four died from transplant complications: graft versus host disease (GvHD), HLH, and severe viral infections.[58]

INFLAMMASOME DISORDERS

Inflammasomes are intracellular multiprotein complexes serving as a key component of the innate immune system. Inflammasomes are responsible for regulating the immunologic response to exogenous and endogenous factors, thereby crucial in protecting the host.[59] The rapid availability of proinflammatory cytokines like IL-1, IL-18, and IL-33 in response to danger signals represents a key mechanism of inflammation. Mutations in 2 of the IL-1 regulating genes, NLRP3 and IL1RN, cause early onset autoinflammatory disease: cryopyrin-associated periodic syndromes (CAPS) and deficiency of IL-1 receptor antagonist (DIRA), respectively.[60] NLRP3 encodes for cryopyrin, an integral part of the cytoplasmic inflammasome. GOF mutations cause activation of the NLRP3 inflammasone, thus upregulating cleavage of inactive pro-IL-1β and pro-IL-18 into their active forms.[60]

Mutations in NLRP3 were first described in 2001 and were associated with familial cold autoinflammatory syndrome (FCAS) and Muckle-Wells syndrome (MWS).[61,62] More recently, NLRP3 mutations were found as the cause of neonatal-onset multisystem inflammatory disease (NOMID). NOMID represents the most severe form of CAPS, characterized by CNS involvement with presence of cerebral calcifications. Thus far, 200 NLRP3 mutations have been reported that lead to CAPS clinical features[63] (**Table 2**). DIRA is caused by autosomal-recessive (AR) biallelic loss-of-function mutations in IL1RN that cause reduced expression of an antagonist of IL-1 signaling, thereby causing overproduction of IL-1β. Disease manifestations occur in the first few weeks of life with overlapping features with CAPS[64] (see **Table 2**).

Three drugs targeting IL-1 have been approved by the US Food and Drug Administration (FDA) for use in the management of CAPS. Anakinra is a short-acting recombinant IL-1 receptor antagonist that blocks both IL-1α and IL-1β binding the IL-1 receptor (see **Table 1**). It is usually given at the doses of 1 to 2 mg/kg subcutaneously

Table 2
Inflammasome disorders treated with interleukin-1 antagonists

	FCAS	MWS	NOMID	DIRA
Gene	*NLRP3*	*NLRP3*	*NLRP3*	*IL1RN*
Inheritance	AD	AD	AD/de novo	AR
Age of onset	Infancy	Infancy-adolescence	Neonatal, infancy	Neonatal
Fever pattern	<24 h	24–48 h	Continuous	Continuous
Cutaneous	Urticarial rash	Urticarial rash	Urticarial rash	Pustular rash Oral mucosal lesions
Neurologic	Conjunctivitis	Conjunctivitis, deafness	Meningitis, deafness, cerebral calcifications	
Musculoskeletal	Arthralgias	Arthralgias	Arthralgias, bony epiphyseal hyperplasia	Arthralgias, periosteal elevation of long bones, widening of ribs and clavicles, multifocal osteolytic lesions
Other			Short stature, frontal bossing, delayed closure of fontanelle	

daily with the maximum dose of 100 mg/d. No serious adverse effect was noted with anakinra use except for an increase in infection risk and injection site reactions. Rilonacept, a fusion protein made of IL-1R1 and IL-1RAcP complexed to the Fc portion of IgG1, acts as a soluble decoy receptor, preventing interaction of IL-1 and its receptor, thereby blocking IL-1 action. Rilonacept binds both IL-1α and IL-1β. Doses of 2.2 mg/kg (maximum 160 mg) given subcutaneously once a week used in CAPS had a long-term safety and tolerability profile. Injection site reactions and elevations in liver transaminase levels are described with rilonacept. Canakinumab can be administered subcutaneously every 8 weeks as it has a long half-life. Dosages used are 2 mg/kg for patients less than 40 kg and 150 mg in patients greater than 40 kg. Adverse effects documented with canakinumab usage are infections, neutropenia, thrombocytopenia, and elevations in liver transaminase levels. The use of these medications in CAPS and DIRA has been widely successful at improving clinical manifestations, inflammatory markers, and frequency of disease episodes.[65–68]

NLCR4 GOF (NLR family CARD domain-containing protein 4) gene mutation causes early onset autoinflammatory syndrome that presents with macrophage activation syndrome (MAS) and enterocolitis.[69,70] NLRC4 is expressed in hematopoietic cells and epithelial cells. The activation of NLRC4 protein causes both caspase-1 and caspase-8 activation and consequent overproduction of proinflammatory cytokines

(IL-18 and IL-1β) that are responsible for increased cell death, also known as pyroptosis.[71-73] Administration of IL-1 inhibitory agents has only been able to partially modulate the disease manifestations in these patients. More recently, therapy with recombinant IL-18 binding protein (tadekinig-alfa) was able to improve disease manifestations in a subject affected by NLRC4 GOF disease.[71] A phase 3 clinical trial (NCT03113760) is currently underway of IL-18 binding protein for treatment of IL-18 driven autoinflammation including NLRC4-MAS or X-linked inhibitor of apoptosis (*XIAP*) deficiency (see **Table 1**). A combination of sirolimus and IL-1 inhibition has been attempted in this disease with the aim of reducing activation of caspase-1 and consequent overproduction of IL-1 and IL-18.[71,74] This combination has shown success in treating these patients and may be beneficial where IL-18 binding protein is not available.

SUMMARY

Understanding of disease mechanisms of primary immunodysregulatory disorders has offered the opportunity to alter the abnormal immune response interfering with mechanism of disease normalizing the immune response. Mechanism-based therapy has been effective at reversing disease-related manifestations in primary immunodysregulatory disorders, offering the most precise therapy to patients.

DISCLOSURE

The authors have nothing to disclose.

REFERENCES

1. Lo B, Abdel-Motal UM. Lessons from CTLA-4 deficiency and checkpoint inhibition. Curr Opin Immunol 2017;49:14–9.
2. Kuehn HS, Ouyang W, Lo B, et al. Immune dysregulation in human subjects with heterozygous germline mutations in CTLA4. Science 2014;345:1623–7.
3. Schubert D, Bode C, Kenefeck R, et al. Autosomal dominant immune dysregulation syndrome in humans with CTLA4 mutations. Nat Med 2014;20:1410–6.
4. Schwab C, Gabrysch A, Olbrich P, et al. Phenotype, penetrance, and treatment of 133 cytotoxic T-lymphocyte antigen 4-insufficient subjects. J Allergy Clin Immunol 2018;142:1932–46.
5. Herrero-Beaumont G, Martinez Calatrava MJ, Castaneda S. Abatacept mechanism of action: concordance with its clinical profile. Reumatol Clin 2012;8:78–83.
6. Lee S, Moon JS, Lee CR, et al. Abatacept alleviates severe autoimmune symptoms in a patient carrying a de novo variant in CTLA-4. J Allergy Clin Immunol 2016;137:327–30.
7. van Leeuwen EM, Cuadrado E, Gerrits AM, et al. Treatment of intracerebral lesions with abatacept in a CTLA4-haploinsufficient patient. J Clin Immunol 2018; 38:464–7.
8. Teachey DT, Greiner R, Seif A, et al. Treatment with sirolimus results in complete responses in patients with autoimmune lymphoproliferative syndrome. Br J Haematol 2009;145:101–6.
9. Navarini AA, Hruz P, Berger CT, et al. Vedolizumab as a successful treatment of CTLA-4-associated autoimmune enterocolitis. J Allergy Clin Immunol 2017;139: 1043–1046 e5.
10. Delmonte OM, Castagnoli R, Calzoni E, et al. Inborn errors of immunity with immune dysregulation: from bench to bedside. Front Pediatr 2019;7:353.

11. Slatter MA, Engelhardt KR, Burroughs LM, et al. Hematopoietic stem cell transplantation for CTLA4 deficiency. J Allergy Clin Immunol 2016;138:615–9.e1.

12. Habibi S, Zaki-Dizaji M, Rafiemanesh H, et al. Clinical, immunologic, and molecular spectrum of patients with LPS-responsive beige-like anchor protein deficiency: a systematic review. J Allergy Clin Immunol Pract 2019;7:2379–86.e5.

13. Alkhairy OK, Abolhassani H, Rezaei N, et al. Spectrum of phenotypes associated with mutations in LRBA. J Clin Immunol 2016;36:33–45.

14. Lo B, Zhang K, Lu W, et al. Autoimmune disease. Patients with LRBA deficiency show CTLA4 loss and immune dysregulation responsive to abatacept therapy. Science 2015;349:436–40.

15. Lopez-Herrera G, Tampella G, Pan-Hammarstrom Q, et al. Deleterious mutations in LRBA are associated with a syndrome of immune deficiency and autoimmunity. Am J Hum Genet 2012;90:986–1001.

16. Gamez-Diaz L, August D, Stepensky P, et al. The extended phenotype of LPS-responsive beige-like anchor protein (LRBA) deficiency. J Allergy Clin Immunol 2016;137:223–30.

17. Charbonnier LM, Janssen E, Chou J, et al. Regulatory T-cell deficiency and immune dysregulation, polyendocrinopathy, enteropathy, X-linked-like disorder caused by loss-of-function mutations in LRBA. J Allergy Clin Immunol 2015; 135:217–27.

18. Levy E, Stolzenberg MC, Bruneau J, et al. LRBA deficiency with autoimmunity and early onset chronic erosive polyarthritis. Clin Immunol 2016;168:88–93.

19. Bratanic N, Kovac J, Pohar K, et al. Multifocal gastric adenocarcinoma in a patient with LRBA deficiency. Orphanet J Rare Dis 2017;12:131.

20. Kiykim A, Ogulur I, Dursun E, et al. Abatacept as a long-term targeted therapy for LRBA deficiency. J Allergy Clin Immunol Pract 2019;7:2790–800.e15.

21. Leiding JW, Ballow M. Redefining precision medicine in disorders of immune dysregulation. J Allergy Clin Immunol Pract 2019;7:2801–3.

22. Seidel MG, Hirschmugl T, Gamez-Diaz L, et al. Long-term remission after allogeneic hematopoietic stem cell transplantation in LPS-responsive beige-like anchor (LRBA) deficiency. J Allergy Clin Immunol 2015;135:1384–90.e1-8.

23. Tesch VK, Abolhassani H, Shadur B, et al. Long-term outcome of LRBA deficiency in 76 patients after various treatment modalities as evaluated by the immune deficiency and dysregulation activity (IDDA) score. J Allergy Clin Immunol 2020;145(5):1452–63.

24. Coulter TI, Chandra A, Bacon CM, et al. Clinical spectrum and features of activated phosphoinositide 3-kinase delta syndrome: a large patient cohort study. J Allergy Clin Immunol 2017;139:597–606.e4.

25. Angulo I, Vadas O, Garcon F, et al. Phosphoinositide 3-kinase delta gene mutation predisposes to respiratory infection and airway damage. Science 2013;342: 866–71.

26. Lucas CL, Kuehn HS, Zhao F, et al. Dominant-activating germline mutations in the gene encoding the PI(3)K catalytic subunit p110delta result in T cell senescence and human immunodeficiency. Nat Immunol 2014;15:88–97.

27. Elkaim E, Neven B, Bruneau J, et al. Clinical and immunologic phenotype associated with activated phosphoinositide 3-kinase delta syndrome 2: a cohort study. J Allergy Clin Immunol 2016;138:210–8.e9.

28. Coulter TI, Cant AJ. The treatment of activated PI3Kdelta syndrome. Front Immunol 2018;9:2043.

29. Maccari ME, Abolhassani H, Aghamohammadi A, et al. Disease evolution and response to rapamycin in activated phosphoinositide 3-kinase delta syndrome:

The European Society for Immunodeficiencies-Activated Phosphoinositide 3-Kinase delta Syndrome Registry. Front Immunol 2018;9:543.

30. Michalovich D, Nejentsev S. Activated PI3 kinase delta syndrome: from genetics to therapy. Front Immunol 2018;9:369.

31. Bartok B, Boyle DL, Liu Y, et al. PI3 kinase delta is a key regulator of synoviocyte function in rheumatoid arthritis. Am J Pathol 2012;180:1906–16.

32. Cahn A, Hamblin JN, Begg M, et al. Safety, pharmacokinetics and dose-response characteristics of GSK2269557, an inhaled PI3Kdelta inhibitor under development for the treatment of COPD. Pulm Pharmacol Ther 2017;46:69–77.

33. Fruman DA, Rommel C. PI3K and cancer: lessons, challenges and opportunities. Nat Rev Drug Discov 2014;13:140–56.

34. Rao VK, Webster S, Dalm V, et al. Effective "activated PI3Kdelta syndrome"-targeted therapy with the PI3Kdelta inhibitor leniolisib. Blood 2017;130:2307–16.

35. Gopal AK, Kahl BS, de Vos S, et al. PI3Kdelta inhibition by idelalisib in patients with relapsed indolent lymphoma. N Engl J Med 2014;370:1008–18.

36. Nademi Z, Slatter MA, Dvorak CC, et al. Hematopoietic stem cell transplant in patients with activated PI3K delta syndrome. J Allergy Clin Immunol 2017;139:1046–9.

37. Villarino AV, Kanno Y, Ferdinand JR, et al. Mechanisms of Jak/STAT signaling in immunity and disease. J Immunol 2015;194:21–7.

38. Casanova JL, Holland SM, Notarangelo LD. Inborn errors of human JAKs and STATs. Immunity 2012;36:515–28.

39. Vargas-Hernandez A, Witalisz-Siepracka A, Prchal-Murphy M, et al. Human signal transducer and activator of transcription 5b (STAT5b) mutation causes dysregulated human natural killer cell maturation and impaired lytic function. J Allergy Clin Immunol 2020;145:345–57.e9.

40. Sampaio EP, Hsu AP, Pechacek J, et al. Signal transducer and activator of transcription 1 (STAT1) gain-of-function mutations and disseminated coccidioidomycosis and histoplasmosis. J Allergy Clin Immunol 2013;131:1624–34.

41. Zhang Y, Ma CA, Lawrence MG, et al. PD-L1 up-regulation restrains Th17 cell differentiation in STAT3 loss- and STAT1 gain-of-function patients. J Exp Med 2017;214:2523–33.

42. Liu L, Okada S, Kong XF, et al. Gain-of-function human STAT1 mutations impair IL-17 immunity and underlie chronic mucocutaneous candidiasis. J Exp Med 2011;208:1635–48.

43. Toubiana J, Okada S, Hiller J, et al. Heterozygous STAT1 gain-of-function mutations underlie an unexpectedly broad clinical phenotype. Blood 2016;127:3154–64.

44. van de Veerdonk FL, Plantinga TS, Hoischen A, et al. STAT1 mutations in autosomal dominant chronic mucocutaneous candidiasis. N Engl J Med 2011;365:54–61.

45. Pedraza-Sanchez S, Lezana-Fernandez JL, Gonzalez Y, et al. Disseminated tuberculosis and chronic mucocutaneous candidiasis in a patient with a gain-of-function mutation in signal transduction and activator of transcription 1. Front Immunol 2017;8:1651.

46. Uzel G, Sampaio EP, Lawrence MG, et al. Dominant gain-of-function STAT1 mutations in FOXP3 wild-type immune dysregulation-polyendocrinopathy-enteropathy-X-linked-like syndrome. J Allergy Clin Immunol 2013;131:1611–23.

47. Vargas-Hernandez A, Mace EM, Zimmerman O, et al. Ruxolitinib partially reverses functional natural killer cell deficiency in patients with signal transducer

and activator of transcription 1 (STAT1) gain-of-function mutations. J Allergy Clin Immunol 2018;141:2142–55.e5.

48. Leiding JW, Okada S, Hagin D, et al. Hematopoietic stem cell transplantation in patients with gain-of-function signal transducer and activator of transcription 1 mutations. J Allergy Clin Immunol 2018;141:704–17.e5.

49. Forbes LR, Vogel TP, Cooper MA, et al. Jakinibs for the treatment of immune dysregulation in patients with gain-of-function signal transducer and activator of transcription 1 (STAT1) or STAT3 mutations. J Allergy Clin Immunol 2018;142:1665–9.

50. Leiding JW, Forbes LR. Mechanism-based precision therapy for the treatment of primary immunodeficiency and primary immunodysregulatory diseases. J Allergy Clin Immunol Pract 2019;7:761–73.

51. Weinacht KG, Charbonnier LM, Alroqi F, et al. Ruxolitinib reverses dysregulated T helper cell responses and controls autoimmunity caused by a novel signal transducer and activator of transcription 1 (STAT1) gain-of-function mutation. J Allergy Clin Immunol 2017;139:1629–40.e2.

52. Chaudhry A, Rudra D, Treuting P, et al. CD4+ regulatory T cells control TH17 responses in a STAT3-dependent manner. Science 2009;326:986–91.

53. Flanagan SE, Haapaniemi E, Russell MA, et al. Activating germline mutations in STAT3 cause early-onset multi-organ autoimmune disease. Nat Genet 2014;46:812–4.

54. Harris TJ, Grosso JF, Yen HR, et al. Cutting edge: An in vivo requirement for STAT3 signaling in TH17 development and TH17-dependent autoimmunity. J Immunol 2007;179:4313–7.

55. Haddad E. STAT3: too much may be worse than not enough! Blood 2015;125:583–4.

56. Haapaniemi EM, Kaustio M, Rajala HL, et al. Autoimmunity, hypogammaglobulinemia, lymphoproliferation, and mycobacterial disease in patients with activating mutations in STAT3. Blood 2015;125:639–48.

57. Milner JD, Vogel TP, Forbes L, et al. Early-onset lymphoproliferation and autoimmunity caused by germline STAT3 gain-of-function mutations. Blood 2015;125:591–9.

58. Fabre A, Marchal S, Barlogis V, et al. Clinical Aspects of STAT3 gain-of-function germline mutations: a systematic review. J Allergy Clin Immunol Pract 2019;7:1958–69.e9.

59. Sonmez HE, Ozen S. A clinical update on inflammasomopathies. Int Immunol 2017;29:393–400.

60. Martinon F, Burns K, Tschopp J. The inflammasome: a molecular platform triggering activation of inflammatory caspases and processing of proIL-beta. Mol Cell 2002;10:417–26.

61. Hoffman HM, Mueller JL, Broide DH, et al. Mutation of a new gene encoding a putative pyrin-like protein causes familial cold autoinflammatory syndrome and Muckle-Wells syndrome. Nat Genet 2001;29:301–5.

62. Cuisset L, Drenth JP, Berthelot JM, et al. Genetic linkage of the Muckle-Wells syndrome to chromosome 1q44. Am J Hum Genet 1999;65:1054–9.

63. Feldmann J, Prieur AM, Quartier P, et al. Chronic infantile neurological cutaneous and articular syndrome is caused by mutations in CIAS1, a gene highly expressed in polymorphonuclear cells and chondrocytes. Am J Hum Genet 2002;71:198–203.

64. Aksentijevich I, Masters SL, Ferguson PJ, et al. An autoinflammatory disease with deficiency of the interleukin-1-receptor antagonist. N Engl J Med 2009;360:2426–37.

65. Hoffman HM, Rosengren S, Boyle DL, et al. Prevention of cold-associated acute inflammation in familial cold autoinflammatory syndrome by interleukin-1 receptor antagonist. Lancet 2004;364:1779–85.

66. Hoffman HM, Throne ML, Amar NJ, et al. Efficacy and safety of rilonacept (interleukin-1 Trap) in patients with cryopyrin-associated periodic syndromes: results from two sequential placebo-controlled studies. Arthritis Rheum 2008;58: 2443–52.

67. Goldbach-Mansky R, Dailey NJ, Canna SW, et al. Neonatal-onset multisystem inflammatory disease responsive to interleukin-1beta inhibition. N Engl J Med 2006; 355:581–92.

68. Lachmann HJ, Kone-Paut I, Kuemmerle-Deschner JB, et al. Use of canakinumab in the cryopyrin-associated periodic syndrome. N Engl J Med 2009;360:2416–25.

69. Alcazar R, Garcia AV, Kronholm I, et al. Natural variation at Strubbelig receptor kinase 3 drives immune-triggered incompatibilities between arabidopsis thaliana accessions. Nat Genet 2010;42:1135–9.

70. Canna SW, de Jesus AA, Gouni S, et al. An activating NLRC4 inflammasome mutation causes autoinflammation with recurrent macrophage activation syndrome. Nat Genet 2014;46:1140–6.

71. Canna SW, Girard C, Malle L, et al. Life-threatening NLRC4-associated hyperinflammation successfully treated with IL-18 inhibition. J Allergy Clin Immunol 2017; 139:1698–701.

72. Romberg N, Vogel TP, Canna SW. NLRC4 inflammasomopathies. Curr Opin Allergy Clin Immunol 2017;17:398–404.

73. Romberg N, Al Moussawi K, Nelson-Williams C, et al. Mutation of NLRC4 causes a syndrome of enterocolitis and autoinflammation. Nat Genet 2014;46:1135–9.

74. Barsalou J, Blincoe A, Fernandez I, et al. Rapamycin as an adjunctive therapy for NLRC4 associated macrophage activation syndrome. Front Immunol 2018;9: 2162.

Nuts and Bolts of Subcutaneous Therapy

Carla Duff, CPNP-PC, MSN, APRN, IgCN[a], Mark Ballow, MD[b],*

KEYWORDS

- SCIG • Immune deficiency • Immunoglobulin replacement therapy
- Subcutaneous infusion

KEY POINTS

- Immunoglobulin replacement therapy is standard of care for humoral immunodeficiencies characterized by impaired antibody production.
- Currently, patients have the choice of IVIG, SCIG, or f-SCIG as therapy options.
- SCIG is as efficacious as IVIG and has multiple clinical advantages including less systemic adverse events and no need for venous access.

INTRODUCTION

Immunoglobulin replacement therapy is the standard of care in treatment of many primary immunodeficiency diseases, especially those with common variable immunodeficiency, hypogammaglobulinemia, and/or antibody deficiency. Immunoglobulin replacement therapy is most often lifelong, therefore ease of administration is vital for adherence to treatment. Immunoglobulin replacement therapy was first used in 1952 when Colonel Ogden Bruton administered immunoglobulin therapy via subcutaneous infusion to a boy with agammaglobulinemia. Bruton was then able to determine that when the immunoglobulin level was detectable, the frequency and severity of infections decreased.[1] Intramuscular immunoglobulin therapy, available since the 1960s, was extremely painful and administering large enough doses to protect from infection was difficult. Intravenous immunoglobulin (IVIG) became widely available in the 1980s, which facilitated larger treatment doses and reduced the pain and trauma of treatment. Subcutaneous intravenous immunoglobulin (SCIG) was later used by Berger and colleagues in the 1980s and its widespread use was described in Europe in 1991.[2–4] In 2006, the first product specifically licensed for SCIG was approved in the United States. In 2014, facilitated SCIG (f-SCIG) composed

[a] Department of Allergy and Immunology, College of Medicine, College of Nursing, University of South Florida, 601 5th Street South, St Petersburg, FL 33701, USA; [b] Division of Allergy and Immunology, Department of Pediatrics, Children's Research Institute, University of South Florida, Johns Hopkins All Children's Hospital, 140 7th Avenue South, CRI 4008, St Petersburg, FL 33701, USA
* Corresponding author.
E-mail address: mballow@usf.edu

Immunol Allergy Clin N Am 40 (2020) 527–537
https://doi.org/10.1016/j.iac.2020.04.002
0889-8561/20/© 2020 Elsevier Inc. All rights reserved.

of two components, human recombinant hyaluronidase (administered first to open up the subcutaneous spaces temporarily) and Gammagard 10% (infused within 10 minutes), was approved for use in adults in the United States. The dosing, processing of immunoglobulin, and route of administration have evolved over the last six decades.

IVIG is an effective method of treatment, most often given every 3 to 4 weeks. However, some patients experience systemic side effects; rise and fall of IgG levels, which has been associated with malaise; and difficult intravenous (IV) access. Traditional SCIG is equally effective with smaller doses administered daily to every 2 weeks, depending on the product. SCIG is associated with fewer systemic side effects yet local site reactions are common. f-SCIG is equally efficacious, and is typically administered every 3 to 4 weeks. With f-SCIG patients must first administer hyaluronidase and then infuse the gammaglobulin. Some 10% IVIG products have been Food and Drug Administration–approved to be given subcutaneously, but 16% and 20% SCIG products are designed to be administered subcutaneously only.

SUBCUTANEOUS INTRAVENOUS IMMUNOGLOBULIN VERSUS INTRAVENOUS IMMUNOGLOBULIN

Immediately after an IVIG infusion, the IgG level increases two-fold or more. The average half-life of IVIG is 21 days, thus IVIG is typically given every 3 or 4 weeks. During this time, the immunoglobulin concentrations vary by 250% to 300% from the peak to the trough.[5] SCIG doses are a fraction of the monthly IVIG dose and thus the peaks and troughs are not so varied. This results in a constant (steady state) serum IgG level (**Fig. 1**). f-SCIG is designed to be administered every 3 to 4 weeks and has a less drastic peak with a trough IgG level similar to IVIG (**Fig. 2**).

In clinical trials, efficacy has been measured by the incidence of acute serious bacterial infections per year.[6] Per the Food and Drug Administration regulations, these infections include bacteremia sepsis, pneumonia, visceral abscess, osteomyelitis or septic arthritis, and bacterial meningitis. The minimal criteria for licensing an immunoglobulin product is a mean of less than 1.0 acute serious bacterial infections per patient-year.

Studies suggest that SCIG is equally efficacious to IVIG even though there have been no direct comparison studies.[6] Meta-analysis of both routes of administration led to similar conclusions that no plateau effect is noted in immunoglobulin levels or in the decreased incidence of infections in relation to doses up to 1 g/kg/mo.[7] Some studies

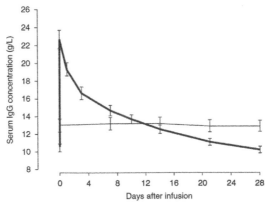

Fig. 1. Subcutaneous and intravenous serum immunoglobulin levels. (*Adapted from* Berger M. Subcutaneous immunoglobulin replacement in primary immunodeficiencies. Clin Immunol 2004;112(1):4; with permission.)

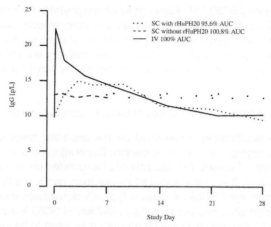

Fig. 2. Kinetics of serum IgG levels. AUC, area under the curve. (*From* Wasserman RL, Melamed I, Stein MR, et al. Recombinant human hyaluronidase-facilitated subcutaneous infusion of human immunoglobulins for primary immunodeficiency. J Allergy Clin Immunol 2012;130(4):954 e11; with permission.)

suggest that the steady-state IgG level achieved with SCIG may better protect against infections because the small, consistent dose delivery mimics the body's antibody production.[2] Immunoglobulin replacement therapy is typically dosed according to body weight and retrospective research studies support this dosing method.[8]

With respect to viral transmission safety, SCIG and IVIG are generally equivalent. Safety in this instance refers to the lack of disease transmission.[5] Immunoglobulin products available in the United States are made from plasma collected from donors in the United States. This plasma is then carefully screened and each product manufacturer carries out procedures to inactivate or remove viruses.[9] There are no reported cases of viruses transmitted by SCIG and none for IVIG since 1994.[10]

Thrombotic events are rare but have been reported with IVIG and SCIG. These rare events, occurring in approximately 0.1% of patients receiving treatment, occur more often with high dosages, more rapid infusions, and underlying risk factors that predispose to thrombosis. Thrombotic events are thought to occur because of an activated clotting factor XIa, a contaminant present in varying degrees in immunoglobulin products.[5]

Another complication reported in IVIG and SCIG is hemolysis, although it occurs more frequently with IVIG in patients receiving large doses for the treatment of autoimmune disorders. Hemolysis is estimated to occur in 1:10,000 infusions. Subsequent anemia may be severe enough to require a transfusion. Hemolysis is caused by isoagglutinins present in immunoglobulin. Current standards require isoagglutinin titers of less than 1:64.[5] Risk factors for hemolysis include preexisting hemolytic disease, inflammatory states, and rapid high-dose infusions.

The tolerability or adverse events with SCIG and IVIG differ. About 10% to 25% of patients receiving IVIG have mild systemic reactions including headache, back pain, and malaise and about 5% of patients have severe systemic adverse events. Systemic adverse events are rare in patients receiving SCIG. This is likely caused by slower absorption of the IgG. However, local site reactions are common with at least 80% of patients reporting site reactions with the first infusion. Local reactions decrease to 30% with subsequent infusions. Site reactions or local reactions are similar with f-SCIG and SCIG. However, f-SCIG has more systemic side effects than SCIG. There are also no reported cases of anaphylaxis with SCIG. In fact, patients that have had anaphylaxis with IVIG have tolerated SCIG.[11,12] Rare cases of anaphylaxis with IVIG have been reported in association with IgE anti-IgA antibodies in patients with IgA deficiency. SCIG and IVIG contain warning labels regarding the use in patient with anti-IgA antibodies.[5] In comparison with IV administration, subcutaneous delivery is increasingly becoming the preferred route of delivery for many patients because of its flexibility and mitigation of side effects.[13]

SUBCUTANEOUS INTRAVENOUS IMMUNOGLOBULIN DOSING AND INFUSION

The dose of SCIG is ultimately determined by the provider; however, most patients receive 400 to 600 mg/kg over a 4-week period. Depending on the product, this dose is divided daily to every 2 weeks. The dose should be rounded up or down to the nearest vial size or the infusion frequency adjusted rather than use a fraction of a dose and discard the remainder. For f-SCIG the dose is typically administered every 3 to 4 weeks via one or two infusion sites. Because the bioavailability of SCIG is about two-thirds the dose administered IV, the monthly infusion amount may need to be increased by a factor of approximately 1.3. However, many providers prefer to use the same dose that was given IV (1:1 dosing). Volume per infusion site and frequency of dosing is decided by the provider based on the tolerability of the patient and recommendations in the package insert.[2] Per the package inserts, patients should receive a loading dose of IVIG before beginning SCIG therapy to ensure an adequate and therapeutic immunoglobulin level. A typical loading dose is 400 to 600 mg/kg via IV followed by the first SCIG 1 week after the last IVIG. The first SCIG dose should be administered within 1 week of the IVIG loading dose. If preferred, patients may receive smaller doses of SCIG consecutively for 3 to 5 days and then begin replacement SCIG dose within 1 week. Patients may need different IgG levels to remain clinically well and infection free. Thus, dosing must be individualized to achieve the maximum clinical outcome.[14] Dose adjustments may also be necessary for weight gain, pregnancy, or significant weight loss.

There are a variety of SCIG products available for commercial use. Products range from 10% to 20% concentration. The choice of SCIG product is usually determined by the provider in conjunction with the patient. The volume to be infused depends on the concentration of the product. For example, 10 g of a 10% product is 100 mL, whereas 10 g of a 20% product is 50 mL. The number of infusion sites is often dependent on the total volume to be infused.[2]

Next are some examples of optimizing and individualizing SCIG therapy:

1. A 10-kg child is beginning SCIG at a dose of 4 g monthly. This dose could be given as 1 g every week or 2 g every 2 weeks. It would be difficult to give this dose every 5 or 10 days because of vial size. Remember, dose should be rounded up or down to nearest vial size.
2. A 40-kg patient is on IVIG and wants to transition to SCIG. The current dose is 20 g monthly. You decide to dose SCIG at 1:1 (IVIG dose/SCIG dose) dosing. This could be given as 5 g weekly, 4 g every 5 days, 7 g every 10 days, or 10 g every 2 weeks. Consideration for number of infusion sites and volume may be dependent on the product concentration, patient body mass index, and patient preference.
3. An 80-kg adult is receiving IVIG 40 g every 3 weeks (roughly 50 g monthly) and wishes to switch to SCIG because of systematic adverse events. Using 1:1 SCIG dosing, the patient can receive 12 g weekly, 6 g every 5 days, 15 g every 10 days, or 25 g biweekly. Keep in mind dose may need to be adjusted based on clinical outcomes and IgG levels.
4. A 70-kg adult is receiving SCIG 10 g weekly and wants to begin daily infusions. This patient could receive 2 g daily Monday through Friday, or 1 g Monday through

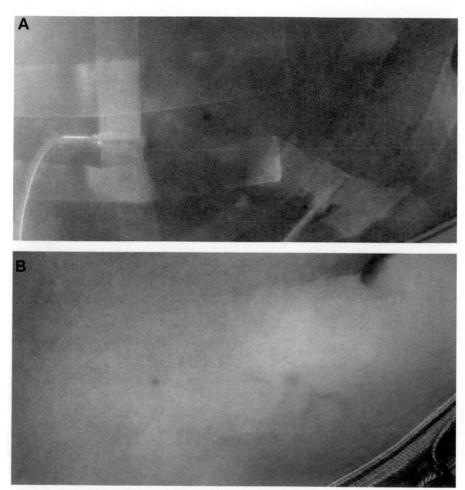

Fig. 3. Site reactions. Mild erythema and swelling (*A*) during and (*B*) immediately after SCIG infusion. (*Courtesy of* C. Duff, CPNP-PC, MSN, APRN, IgCN, St. Petersburg, FL.)

Friday and 5 g on Saturday, or 2 g Monday through Wednesday and 1 g Thursday through Sunday.

The key to achieving an optimal and individualized SCIG therapy regimen is flexibility. Discuss with the patient the number of days they want to infuse and the volume and number of sites they wish to use; then create an infusion regimen that fits into their lifestyle and for which they can be compliant.

Infusion site reactions are common and improve over time. Some patients may develop swelling without erythema or vice versa. The swelling and erythema typically resolve within 24 hours postinfusion and after 72 hours it is difficult to determine the location of the site of infusion. Patients who have received SCIG for years do not have changes in the tissue based on examination.[5] However, some patients do develop hard nodules at the infusion site that dissipate over time spontaneously. Patients have reported redness, itching, and leaking at the insertion site and discomfort with the needle and prolonged infusion time (**Figs. 3** and **4**). Troubleshooting site reactions (**Table 1**) can ease the patient's discomfort and improve their infusion

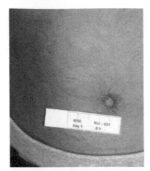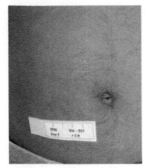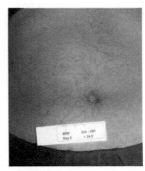

Fig. 4. Subcutaneous infusion. 0 minutes postinfusion, 8 hours postinfusion, and 24 hours postinfusion. (© CSL Behring LLC; used by permission; all rights reserved.)

experience. Often times, adjusting or changing ancillary supplies resolves the issues with site reactions (**Fig. 5**).

There are multiple sites commonly used for SCIG infusions (**Fig. 6**). Most commonly used are the abdomen, thigh, flank, buttocks, and upper arm. Patients should be instructed to stay 2 inches away from their umbilicus, scar tissue, striae, and other

Table 1
Troubleshooting SCIG site reactions

Injection-site reaction Blanching Redness/rash Itching Discomfort Swelling	Assess for tape allergy; change to paper/hypoallergenic tape Assess size; choose a needle size that is consistent with volume being infused Assess length of catheter; may be too short and fluid may be leaking into intradermal layer Assess site location; may be too close to muscle Decrease rate of infusion or decease volume per site Avoid tracking IgG through the intradermal tissue by not allowing drops of IgG on needle tip before needle insertion Assess appropriateness of rotating sites Consider use of topical anesthetic ointment
Leaking at catheter site	Assess catheter; ensure it is affixed securely and fully inserted Assess placement; may be in location that is subject to movement; advise regarding selection of site Assess length of catheter; may be too short; suggest change Assess infusion volume; amount per site may be too great; adjust volume Assess rate of infusion; adjust rate
Extreme discomfort with needle	Assess needle length; may be too long and irritating abdominal wall Try catheter that allows introducer needle to be removed, leaving indwelling flexible cannula catheter Try ice or topical anesthetic cream before insertion
Long infusion time	Assess infusion preparation; use at room temperature Assess volume per site, rate of infusion, and number of sites, or adjust infusion regimen Check equipment for pump setting, correct selection of tubing size and length to match infusion rates; check pump function, battery function, and so forth Arrange observation of patient technique (specialty pharmacy provider or office visit)
Blood return observed	Remove and discard catheter that demonstrated blood return; use new set (notify supplier of need for replacement)

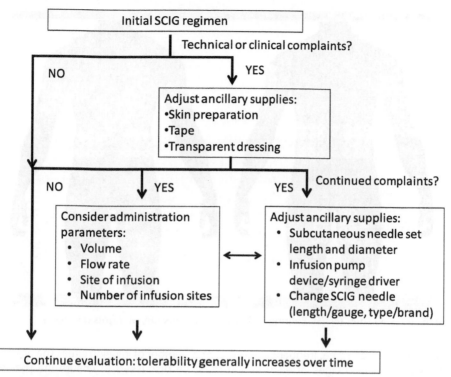

Fig. 5. Treatment algorithm for patients with technical or clinical complaints during or following initial SCIG regimen. (*From* Duff C, Ochoa D, Riley P, et al. Importance of ancillary supplies for subcutaneous immunoglobulin infusion: management of the local infusion site. J Infus Nurs 2013;36(6):388; with permission.)

infusion sites. The number of sites varies per patient depending on body mass, volume to be infused, and infusion rate. A slender individual may need more infusion sites because they may not tolerate a large volume per site. A patient with more body mass may tolerate a much larger volume per site. Depending on the product, 25 to 60 mL may be infused per site (see package insert) based on patient tolerability. For a small volume, the dose may infuse rapidly in 15 to 30 minutes. For a larger dose, the infusion time is slower, often 1 hour or more.

SCIG is appropriate for all ages, from neonates to the elderly. SCIG has not been studied in licensing trails for children less than 2 years of age but many publications indicate it is safe and effective for this age group. Currently, f-SCIG is licensed for adult use only. SCIG may be preferable in children and the elderly because IV access is not required. Administration of f-SCIG is more complicated using a different process because of the two-drug regimen and different types of tubing and pumps needed for the infusion. To ensure success and compliance with infusions, the SCIG regimen (frequency, infusion volume, infusion rate, and selection site) must be optimized for the best clinical outcome.

INITIATING SUBCUTANEOUS INTRAVENOUS IMMUNOGLOBULIN THERAPY

The decision to treat primary immune deficiency with SCIG must be made jointly between the provider and the patient. It must be a frank and open discussion regarding

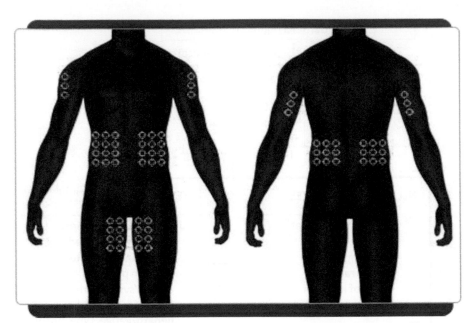

Fig. 6. Infusion sites. (© CSL Behring LLC; used by permission; all rights reserved.)

choice of product, route, frequency, volume, and number of infusion sites. The advantages and disadvantages of each option must be discussed to ensure the patient makes an educated and informed decision. Research indicates that when patients are part of the decision-making process, they are more likely to be compliant and thus have a positive outcome.[15,16]

Before initiating SCIG therapy, the patient must be informed of the benefits and risks associated with immunoglobulin replacement therapy and subcutaneous infusions. All immunoglobulin products have warnings, such as aseptic meningitis, renal impairment, and thrombotic events, and these warnings need to be discussed with patients before beginning therapy. f-SCIG has additional warnings that should also be discussed with patients considering this therapy. Discussion of the benefits, risks, and warnings allow patients to make an informed decision regarding their therapy. Although administration of SCIG is not a difficult process, multiple variables need to be considered and patients' input regarding their therapy must be considered.

For patients to achieve the best possible outcome, a discussion regarding expectations must occur. It is vital for the patient to have realistic expectations regarding their SCIG infusion. These expectations include necessary equipment, supplies, instructions for administration, and common side effects including local site reactions and effectiveness of therapy. Patients must also be educated as to when they will notice a difference in their symptoms post-therapy. Often, patients think one infusion will make them better. Patients must also understand that although the goal of immunoglobulin therapy is to reduce the severity and frequency of infections, immunoglobulin replacement therapy does not prevent all infections. Patients with realistic expectations tend to be have better outcomes and improved compliancy.[15,17]

An educated, trained, and experienced nurse provides the SCIG teaching for the patient. During these teach and train sessions, the patient is educated on infusions preparation, pump set up, administration, infusion techniques, and supply disposal. **(Table 2)** The patient should be provided with an infusion check list and contact

Table 2 Procedure for administration of SCIG	
Step 1	Wash hands. This procedure is aseptic and not sterile. Gloves are not required for self-infusion.
Step 2	Assemble supplies (pump, medication, tubing, syringe, transfer device, alcohol pads, tape, and gauze or band aids) on a clean surface. Wash surface, such as countertop, with soap and water or use an alcohol pad.
Step 3	Examine the medications and ensure it is not expired. The vial should be clear with nothing floating in it. If vials are expired or otherwise unusable, contact specialty pharmacy.
Step 4	Using the syringe and transfer device, draw up the medication. Patent should be trained to use the entire vial. Depending on the dose, more than 1 syringe may be required.
Step 5	Prime the tubing but do not allow the medication to reach the needle. There is no concern if there is air or bubbles in the line because this infusion is subcutaneous.
Step 6	Choose and clean the infusion site. Infusion sites should be 2 inches apart. Scars and striae should be avoided.
Step 7	Insert the needle at a 90-degree angle into the site and secure.
Step 8	Turn on the pump and begin infusion. Depending on the pump, an Infusion rate may need to be programmed.
Step 9	Infusion complete. Turn off pump. Withdrawal needle. Dispose of supplies. Complete infusion diary.

numbers. The nurse goes through each step of the infusion process and the patient must demonstrate proficiency at every step. Once the patient demonstrates proficiency they will administer their SCIG in their home on their own schedule. A health care professional will no longer be required to be present for each infusion. However, should the patient encounter difficulties with their infusion, a follow-up visit to troubleshoot issues is arranged. This may require that ancillary supplies be changed.[18–28] There is a variety of educational materials available for the patient and the health care provider to ensure the success of SCIG infusions (See **Table 1**).

Once a patient has been trained and is self-administering SCIG, the provider must discuss SCIG infusions at each visit. This is to ensure that the patient continues to infuse properly with as few adverse reactions as possible. IgG levels must continue to be monitored and if necessary, the dose of SCIG adjusted to maintain a therapeutic level. Discussing the infusion and monitoring laboratory data help to ensure compliance.

SUMMARY

Immunoglobulin replacement therapy is standard of care for humoral immunodeficiencies characterized by impaired antibody production. Because these diseases are lifelong with no known cure, patients who receive immunoglobulin therapy often do so for life. Thus, choosing the best therapy option for each patient is vital to their long-term health outcomes. Currently, patients have the choice of IVIG, SCIG, or f-SCIG as therapy options. Many variables including disease, comorbidities, and patient lifestyle must be considered when choosing which therapy option is best for each patient. For many patients SCIG is the preferred option. SCIG is as efficacious as IVIG and has multiple clinical advantages including less systemic adverse events and no need for venous access. Because SCIG is self-administered in the patient home, there is no need for an infusion appointment and instead patients have the flexibility and autonomy to manage their infusions on their own. However, this independence and autonomy does increase patient responsibility. SCIG also allows patient input to design their own individualized and optimal treatment plan. Because SCIG regimens are flexible and allow for increased autonomy, patients receiving SCIG report an improved quality of life.[2] As providers, our role in ensuing success of SCIG therapy with proper education, training, and support for the patient is vital.

DISCLOSURE

C. Duff: CSL Behring, nurse consultant; Takeda, presenter; Grifols, nurse consultant. M. Ballow: physician advisory board and speaker bureau for CSL Behring, Takeda, and Grifols; consulting medical director for the Immune Deficiency Foundation; Data Safety Monitoring Board, Prometic, Glenmark.

REFERENCES

1. Khan WN. Colonel Bruton's kinase defined the molecular basis of X-linked agammaglobulinemia, the first primary immunodeficiency. J Immunol 2012;188(7): 2933–5.
2. Younger ME, Blouin W, Duff C, et al. Subcutaneous immunoglobulin replacement therapy: ensuring success. J Infus Nurs 2015;38(1):70–9.
3. New immune globulin product. FDA Consumer 2006;40(2):2.
4. Guidance for industry: safety, efficacy, and pharmacokinetic studies to support marketing of immune globulin intravenous (human) as replacement therapy for primary humoral immunodeficiency. U.S. Department of Health and Human Services Food and Drug Administration Center for Biologics Evaluation and Research (CBER); 2008. Available at: http://www.fda.gov/biologicsbloodvaccines/guidancecomplianceregulatoryinformation/guidances/blood/ucm072130.htm. Accessed July 1, 2014.
5. Francisco A, Duff C. In focus: subcutaneous immunoglobulin (SCIG). Towson, Maryland: An Immune Deficient Foundation (IDF) Publication; 2015.
6. Berger M. Subcutaneous immunoglobulin replacement in primary immunodeficiencies. Clin Immunol 2004;112(1):1–7.
7. Orange JS, Belohradsky BH, Berger M, et al. Evaluation of correlation between dose and clinical outcomes in subcutaneous immunoglobulin replacement therapy. Clin Exp Immunol 2012;169(2):172–81.
8. Shapiro R. Subcutaneous immunoglobulin (16 or 20%) therapy in obese patients with primary immunodeficiency: a retrospective analysis of administration by infusion pump or subcutaneous rapid push. Clin Exp Immunol 2013;173(2):365–71.
9. Hooper JA. Intravenous immunoglobulins: evolution of commercial IVIG preparations. Immunol Allergy Clin N Am 2008;28(4):765–78, viii.
10. Siegel J. Safety considerations in IGIV utilization. Int Immunopharmacol 2006; 6(4):523–7.
11. Rachid R, Bonilla FA. The role of anti-IgA antibodies in causing adverse reactions to gamma globulin infusion in immunodeficient patients: a comprehensive review of the literature. J Allergy Clin Immunol 2012;129(3):628–34.

12. Horn J, Thon V, Bartonkova D, et al. Anti-IgA antibodies in common variable immunodeficiency (CVID): diagnostic workup and therapeutic strategy. Clin Immunol 2007;122(2):156–62.
13. Shapiro RS. Subcutaneous immunoglobulin therapy given by subcutaneous rapid push vs infusion pump: a retrospective analysis. Ann Allergy Asthma Immunol 2013;111(1):51–5.
14. Ballow M. Practical aspects of immunoglobulin replacement. Ann Allergy Asthma Immunol 2017;119(4):299–303.
15. Samaan K, Levasseur MC, Decaluwe H, et al. SCIg vs. IVIg: let's give patients the choice! J Clin Immunol 2014;34(6):611–4.
16. Burton J, Murphy E, Riley P. Primary immunodeficiency disease: a model for case management of chronic diseases. Prof Case Manag 2010;15(1):5–10, 2-4; [quiz: 5-6].
17. Younger ME, Aro L, Blouin W, et al. Nursing guidelines for administration of immunoglobulin replacement therapy. J infusion Nurs 2013;36(1):58–68.
18. Duff C, Ochoa D, Riley P, et al. Importance of ancillary supplies for subcutaneous immunoglobulin infusion: management of the local infusion site. J infusion Nurs 2013;36(6):384–90.
19. Orange JS, Grossman WJ, Navickis RJ, et al. Impact of trough IgG on pneumonia incidence in primary immunodeficiency: a meta-analysis of clinical studies. Clin Immunol 2010;137(1):21–30.
20. Burks AW, Sampson HA, Buckley RH. Anaphylactic reactions after gamma globulin administration in patients with hypogammaglobulinemia. Detection of IgE antibodies to IgA. N Engl J Med 1986;314(9):560–4.
21. Menis M, Sridhar G, Selvam N, et al. Hyperimmune globulins and same-day thrombotic adverse events as recorded in a large healthcare database during 2008-2011. Am J Hematol 2013;88(12):1035–40.
22. Sridhar G, Ekezue BF, Izurieta HS, et al. Immune globulins and same-day thrombotic events as recorded in a large health care database during 2008 to 2012. Transfusion 2014;54(10):2553–65.
23. Desborough MJ, Miller J, Thorpe SJ, et al. Intravenous immunoglobulin-induced haemolysis: a case report and review of the literature. Transfus Med 2014;24(4):219–26.
24. Berard R, Whittemore B, Scuccimarri R. Hemolytic anemia following intravenous immunoglobulin therapy in patients treated for Kawasaki disease: a report of 4 cases. Pediatr Rheumatol Online J 2012;10(1):10.
25. Berger M. Adverse effects of IgG therapy. J Allergy Clin Immunol Pract 2013;1(6):558–66.
26. Lingman-Framme J, Fasth A. Subcutaneous immunoglobulin for primary and secondary immunodeficiencies: an evidence-based review. Drugs 2013;73(12):1307.
27. HyQvia. Prescribing information: Baxter. 2015. Available at: http://www.hyqvia.com. Accessed May 1, 2015.
28. Berger M, Jolles S, Orange JS, et al. Bioavailability of IgG administered by the subcutaneous route. J Clin Immunol 2013;33(5):984–90.

Moving?

Make sure your subscription moves with you!

To notify us of your new address, find your **Clinics Account Number** (located on your mailing label above your name), and contact customer service at:

Email: journalscustomerservice-usa@elsevier.com

800-654-2452 (subscribers in the U.S. & Canada)
314-447-8871 (subscribers outside of the U.S. & Canada)

Fax number: 314-447-8029

**Elsevier Health Sciences Division
Subscription Customer Service
3251 Riverport Lane
Maryland Heights, MO 63043**

*To ensure uninterrupted delivery of your subscription, please notify us at least 4 weeks in advance of move.

Printed and bound by CPI Group (UK) Ltd, Croydon, CR0 4YY

03/10/2024

01040405-0010